HIV+
WORKING THE SYSTEM

HIV+

Working the System

by Robert A. Rimer
and Michael A. Connolly

with cartoons by Michael Willhoite

BOSTON: ALYSON PUBLICATIONS, INC.

Published as a trade paperback original by Alyson Publications, Inc., 40 Plympton St., Boston, Mass. 02118.
Distributed in England by GMP Publishers,
P.O. Box 247, London, N17 9QR, England.

First edition, first printing: January 1993.

5 4 3 2 1

ISBN 1-55583-208-3

This book is printed on acid-free, recycled paper.

Library of Congress Cataloging-in-Publication Data

Rimer, Robert A., 1950–
    HIV+ : working the system / by Robert A. Rimer and Michael A. Connolly ; with cartoons by Michael Willhoite. — 1st ed.
        p.   cm.
    ISBN 1-55583-208-3 : $12.95
    1. HIV infections—Popular works.   I. Connolly, Michael A., 1952–
.   II. Title.
RC607.A26R545   1993
362.1'9697'92—dc20   92-30659
                                                                    CIP

Contents

Introduction   9

1   Coping with Ambiguity   15
Question Authority. Living with HIV is ambiguous.
Even the experts will often be wrong.

2   Working the System   43
Understand the HIV bureaucracy by watching all the
moving parts. What you don't know WILL eventually
hurt you.

3   Monitoring Your Health   79
Treat problems empirically. Try simpler things first.

4   Seeking Treatment   101
More medicine is not always better. Treat HIV as a
chronic condition, rather than as a terminal one.

5   Managing Your Doctor   121
Hire a doctor with good administrative skills. Those
skills are the keys to the system.

6   Obtaining Experimental Drugs   153
No one is Running the Show. It's up to you. You are
the only one whose primary objective is to keep you
alive.

7   Reordering Your Priorities   181
Make room in your life for HIV Business. Managing
HIV is your number-one priority.

8   Life Goes On   219

Epilogue: Where Are They Now?   227

Afterword   231

Appendix: Getting More Information   235

Acknowledgments

Thanks to our readers David Aronstein, Ron Cathcart, Bill Kreidler, Jason Schneider, John Smith, and Pat Touzin, for their thoughtful comments, with particular thanks to Jason and Pat who thoroughly critiqued multiple drafts of this book. To Robert Riger, for his expert guidance throughout the entire process. To John LaFauci, who came up with the title. To our cartoonist Michael Willhoite, for his sense of humor. To Rachel, for letting us tell her story. To Kathy McGill and Linda Martyn, for their loving wisdom. To Betty and Joe Revis, for their unwavering support. To Millie and Andre, for the comfort in knowing they are there.

To the staff and volunteers of the AIDS service organizations throughout the country, whom historians will use as examples of real heroes.

We fondly remember Barbara Rimer, Sara Bloom, Nina Hood Brazelton Connolly, Michael Giovinco, Larry Killian, Raymond Dubreuil, and Bob Anderson.

Introduction

My name is Bob Rimer. I was probably infected with HIV before 1980. Since my AIDS diagnosis in 1986, I have been dealing with the HIV system — hospitals, insurance companies, and AIDS service organizations. Living in this bureaucracy with HIV is like living in one grand dysfunctional family. My colleague and friend, Michael Connolly, has joined me in writing this guide to working the HIV system. Although HIV-negative himself, Michael has professional experience with HIV. He is an AIDS activist, and he's personally worked with the HIV system while caring for his lover and friends.

Studies of long-term survivors show that we take control of treatment and our lives. What does that mean? It means asking questions until you get answers that make sense. It means demanding accountability. It means evaluating what's important to you. And it means questioning authority every step of the way.

In my case, I know that *if I'd done as I was told, I'd be dead today.*

That's because our health care bureaucracy has a strong built-in tendency to be unmanageable.

There are two reasons for this. First, doctors view themselves as authority figures; they believe they're smarter than patients, so they expect patients to be compliant. Unfortunately, all too many patients agree. This attitude impedes good two-way communication. Second, the health care system is complex. It has lots of moving parts and little accountability. Consequently, the quality of care is uneven; problems get ignored; people fall through the cracks. Savvy patients, whatever their illness, have long recognized this and sought better care by managing their doctors.

Now HIV is exposing the underlying unmanageability of the health care bureaucracy for all to see.

First, there is the stigma attached to HIV and to the groups afflicted, particularly gay people, blacks, and the poor. This stigma gives insurance companies and other institutions license to snoop on and discriminate against people with HIV. That, in turn, discourages those of us with HIV from communicating openly with our doctors, employers, and support networks.

Then there is the rate of change. The constant development of new treatments makes medical reference materials obsolete almost as soon as they're published. This rate of change is increasing and practitioners don't keep up. Many patients do, however, by approaching activist organizations for information. Neither doctors nor patients are trained to deal with this disparity.

Moreover, medical practitioners are accustomed to treating diseases that have been around a long time. Even when following new procedures for diagnosis and treatment, they're looking *backwards*, because medical procedures are based on studies begun and concluded years ago. For well-researched ailments — measles or diabetes — this perspective often works. For HIV, it does not. Three-year-old data about the treatment of diabetes is still valid. Three-year-old data about HIV is not.

Your best bet today is to treat HIV as a chronic, manageable condition. This approach will improve your quality of life. You'll stay "healthy" longer and you'll live longer. You may well live to see the day when the medical establishment itself proclaims that HIV is a chronic, manageable condition.

Unfortunately, most practitioners still assume that HIV is going to kill you because that's what happened in the past. They don't factor in the continuing development of new treatments. They may overtreat you — or treat you in ways that shut off future treatment options. Therefore, the bottom line is: *People with HIV must manage their practitioners.*

In this book I describe the strategies I've used to stay alive and, incidentally, to have a little fun in the process. It is at once a tour of the HIV system and a storybook — all based on true stories. In many cases, I've used nicknames or pseudonyms to protect the privacy of the individuals concerned, but the dialogue and the details are real.

My mother was mentally ill. She also had cancer. I helped manage her care as I grew up. In so doing, I learned to question doctors and watch the details. Through my exposure to the mental health system, I developed a skeptical attitude and learned to watch out for incompetence. Together with some valuable partners and a good dose of luck, these skills and attitudes have allowed me to survive the HIV system — so far!

My experiences are relevant to people who are living with HIV disease or with any poorly understood life-threatening disease. The system, the emotions, and the spectrum of health issues are basically the same. Left to its own devices, the system will give you outdated care. That was true for people with HIV in 1986; it's still true today; and it will be true tomorrow, in spite of all the new treatments. *To get good care, you must get to know the system and work it.*

Virtually everyone has successfully managed one system or another. We already have system skills. But we get so awed by the doctors, the bureaucrats, and the mind-numbing paperwork that we give away our control. There's an old joke told by both staff and patients in mental hospitals:

Question: What's the difference between the staff and the patients?

Answer: The staff carry the keys!

This book will help you get the keys. I hope you have fun reading it. ■

"Robert has not been conforming
to the rules of the school
or the rules in the classroom."
—Mrs. Walsh;
5th Grade Report Card
Sophia W. Ripley Elementary School
Boston, Massachusetts, 1960

1

Coping with Ambiguity

Y ou don't have AIDS. There's nothing wrong with you."
Dr. Martinez sat back in his chair, stethoscope dan-
gling from his neck, and looked at me sympathetically. It was
November 1985. This was not the first time I received mislead-
ing information. Nor would it be the last.

■

I didn't exactly have a normal upbringing. In fact, Manny and
Barbara should never have had children.

On my first day of kindergarten, Mother forgot to pick me
up. Over time, she lost track of other details.

"What's for dinner, Mummy?" I asked one night when I
was six.

"Mummy cooked dinner *last* night!" she informed me
patiently.

My father's dysfunction was less obvious, but no less real.
When I was eight, during one of my mother's early hospitaliza-
tions, my maternal grandmother would sneak into the house
to leave meals for me and my younger brother, Stephen. One
night when he returned from work, my father, who was not
speaking to his mother-in-law, caught me standing on a stool,
stirring chicken soup. "Has your grandmother been here?" he
said suspiciously.

One summer day, when I was thirteen, Mother took me
and four classmates to the beach. Picture Barbara bombing
up the highway at 85 mph in a nine-passenger Ford station
wagon — while using both hands to tease her hair. Barbara
had invented cruise control way before Ford!

"Mrs. Rimer," said my friend Bernie nervously, "you have
to hold the wheel!"

"All right," she said, resting one hand on the wheel and eyeing her beehive in the mirror. She continued to play with her hair with the other hand. We kept an eye on her for the rest of the trip.

Thus I learned early in life not to uncritically accept everything I was told.

■

Beginning in September 1985, I noticed subtle changes in my health. My energy level seemed off. For ten years, I'd worked out at the gym every other day. Now, I only felt up to working out twice a week — and only for two sets instead of my normal three. Something funny was going on.

In October, a case of food poisoning took me to the Emergency Room at Boston's Beth Israel Hospital, where I was treated by a very nice man — Dr. Martinez. I mentioned I didn't have a doctor and he said, "I'll be your physician." I accepted his offer and scheduled an appointment in November to discuss the changes in my health. An office exam showed no reason for concern. Martinez tried to reassure me. He ordered a battery of blood tests and sent me down to the lab.

On December 1, shortly after my visit to Martinez, I bought a new pair of leather work boots — very butch, I thought, as I put them on later. To my surprise, the left boot was uncomfortable. My foot hurt. I took off the boot and found a bruise on the sole of my foot. A couple weeks later, the bruise was still there. That worried me. I'd heard that spots and bruises were common in people with AIDS.

At the same time, I noticed mucus in my stool, so I went to a public health facility to be tested for syphilis and gonorrhea. The results were negative.

"Something's wrong with me," I said to the nurse.

"All your tests are normal," she replied calmly.

"Okay, but something *is* wrong," I insisted. "My energy level has been off for months. And what is this bruise?"

"Go home and forget about it," she said. "There's nothing wrong with you."

Worried, I scheduled another appointment with Dr. Martinez for early January. "Your November blood test results were fine," he told me. "I'll run them again, but I don't expect any changes." He also found a small spot on my leg, which I had never noticed before.

"Could this be AIDS?" I asked.

"No, that's impossible. Your white count is perfectly normal."

As we walked to the door, he put his hand on my shoulder and said, "Let's just keep an eye on that spot. If it'll make you feel better, you can see a dermatologist."

I should have been reassured, but I wasn't. The medical experts were saying the incubation period for HIV was twelve to twenty-four months. Eighteen months earlier, my lover Mario and I had separated. Afterwards, when seeing other men, I had practiced safer sex, so I thought I was at little risk for AIDS. But I also knew something wasn't right in my body — and it wasn't going away. I started reading about AIDS.

I didn't know anyone with HIV, but I read the newspapers and I'd heard plenty about it from friends in New York. So I bought a book that described the symptoms of AIDS. The author listed night sweats, fevers, diarrhea, and weight loss, as well as spots that won't go away: Kaposi's sarcoma (KS), an AIDS-related cancer. As I read, I got a sinking feeling. The bruise on my foot did not match the description of KS, but the spot on my leg did.

I reviewed all the information. First, my body felt different than it used to. My energy level was lower. Something was wrong. Second, venereal diseases had been ruled out. I'd tested negative. Third, my white blood cell counts were normal. Martinez said that meant no HIV. But he had not tested me for HIV, since he had ruled it out. What if I had AIDS and Martinez didn't know how to diagnose it? I couldn't rule out that possibility.

The situation was ambiguous.

I decided to get another opinion. I called Boston's lesbian and gay community health center and spoke with P. Clay Stevens, a public health counselor.

"I have a spot on my leg that won't go away. My doctor is telling me I can't have AIDS because my white blood cell count is okay. Is it possible I have AIDS?"

"That spot could be serious," she replied. "Your white blood count doesn't mean much. You need to get an HIV test."

I shook my head as I hung up. P. Clay had flatly contradicted my primary care physician. Between what she said and what I'd gleaned from the book, I was really anxious. I called

Dr. Martinez and made an appointment to discuss this contradictory information the following week, which was the
beginning of February.

For days I thought of little else but HIV. Mentally I went
over the information I had. Perhaps the incubation period
was longer than twenty-four months. That would mean I
might have been infected earlier, before safer sex. I might
even have given it to Mario. At night, I saw spots in my
dreams.

A week later, I sat in Martinez's office and looked on as he
leafed through my medical file. He had dark curly hair, a
moustache, and a personable manner. I didn't pick up any
homophobia. I felt he took my concerns seriously, even when
he disagreed with me. I liked him. But I was losing confidence
in his knowledge of HIV.

I began. "The gay health center says you can have AIDS
even if your white count is okay. That spot on my leg is still
there and so is my bruise. This has been going on since September. Now it's February. Shouldn't we do something?"

Until we come up with something else, I thought, *I bet it is
HIV. And the longer we wait, the worse trouble I'll be in.*
Pretending nothing had changed would only increase my
anxiety. It was not an option for me.

"Okay," said Martinez, "I'll humor you. We'll biopsy that
spot. I'll make the appointment."

That evening I drove over to Mario's. After a year-long
separation, we had begun dating again in September. Now we
were planning to move in together. I had already sold my
condo and was about to buy a house in the country. I told
Mario about the bruise and the biopsy appointment — and
said that it might be AIDS. We were both too terrified to talk.
We did start practicing safe sex.

■

My biopsy appointment was at the end of February. I went to
dermatology, extremely anxious. I recited the consequences of
a positive biopsy. *No cure,* I thought. *Stigma, isolation ... no
sex...* I wondered if Mario would still move in with me.

The dermatologist, a dark-haired young woman, looked
me in the eye as I sat down. "So you're here for a biopsy," she
said in a businesslike tone. "Change into a johnny, please."

I undressed anxiously, a lump rising in my throat.

As the doctor examined my leg, I said, "How much do you cut for a biopsy?"

"Not much. I just scrape a bit." She swabbed the spot with alcohol.

"Could this be KS?" I asked.

"We can't tell without doing the biopsy."

"You've seen this stuff before," I continued. "Does it *look* like KS?"

She looked over her glasses at me and responded evenly, "Are you a male homosexual?"

"No," I snorted, "I'm a *female* homosexual!" *Next she'll ask if I'm Haitian,* I thought. She was obviously thinking about the materials she had read on AIDS, in particular the list of what were then called "high-risk groups."

She prepared the specimen container and cut a two-inch gash in my leg.

"How long will it take to get the results?" I asked.

"Three or four days. They'll send them to your primary care doctor. He'll call you." Then I was excused. Procedure over. I felt like a piece of meat.

Four days later, I called Martinez. No results. The next day I called again. Again no results. I continued to call daily from work whenever my officemate, Tom, stepped out.

Tom and I worked for Yankee Atomic, a nuclear power company located off the turnpike west of Boston. I'd left my previous job at a computer consulting firm in the city because I was tired of the stress and the travel. I took the summer off, then came to Yankee on a temp job at fabulous rates. After working a day and a half, I asked for more work. The manager told me, "You just finished a three-week project." Bells went off in my head. Gravy train! Long lunches! Peace and quiet!

Three months later, after I passed a battery of psychological tests and the company shrink had certified me as "sane," they offered me a job. I accepted with some misgivings. The staff was unsophisticated and the culture was very conservative.

My office overlooked the swimming pool of a Sheraton hotel, a mock Tudor castle favored for gaudy weddings. I'll let you imagine, for a moment, what's hanging out around the pool on summer weekdays. Not a pretty sight. As I dialed Martinez, I was drawn to look, nonetheless.

One day, two weeks after my biopsy, Martinez told me, "I got the test back. The results are inconclusive. We're not sure if you have KS."

"You're not sure?" I repeated. "So what are you going to do?"

He hesitated. I could tell he was about to reassure me again. I didn't want reassurance. I wanted information. If it wasn't AIDS, it was something else. "Let's get a conclusive diagnosis. Could you send the biopsy somewhere else, where they can tell?" I asked. "How about New York or San Francisco?"

He consented. Another week passed. I began calling daily again.

On March 21, Martinez finally had news. "Bob, the test results are back." Over three weeks had elapsed since the biopsy.

"Yes? What is it?"

"I'm sorry." He paused. "It's positive. It's KS. Can you come in to see me? We need to talk."

I gazed blankly at the bulletin board, his words ringing in my head. I was shattered.

Tom walked in moments later. I blurted out the news. I had AIDS. I'm not the type to hold something like that in. Then I sought out my manager, Mercedes, and said, "I've just been diagnosed with AIDS. I'm heading in town to see my doctor."

Mercedes was the only woman manager out of eight hundred employees. Other staff had problems with Mercedes, but she and I got along well. Our relationship was professional, but friendly; she knew I was gay.

"But we have a meeting in five minutes!" Mercedes protested weakly. She wasn't even aware of her own denial.

"Well, I'm leaving, Mercedes," I said. I wanted to see Dr. Martinez right away. It would be three weeks before I returned to my office.

An hour later I was in Boston at the hospital. Martinez closed the door behind me and laid his hand on my knee as I settled in the chair, shaking. I was ready for him to flinch or avoid me. He didn't.

"Is there anything I can do for you?" he said hesitantly.

He's crushed, I thought. *He really hadn't anticipated a positive biopsy.* I felt oddly sad for him and concerned.

"Give me a prescription for Valium," I said hoarsely. "I'm going to need it. Today."

"Sure, no problem."

I searched for words. "What's my prognosis?"

"I don't know. I have no idea," he said. He seemed at a loss for words.

"Well, what kind of survival data is there?"

He shook his head. "I'm not sure. I doubt if there's very much."

I drew a deep breath. "How long do I have to live?"

"I don't know."

"Could you make a guess?"

"Nine to twelve months."

To date, Martinez had seen two patients with AIDS. Both were diagnosed when they contracted pneumocystis carinii pneumonia (PCP), an AIDS-related opportunistic infection. They died soon thereafter. Hospitals hadn't yet learned to treat PCP effectively. Now people live through five or six bouts of PCP and most people with HIV forestall it by taking preventive medicine ("prophylaxis," as they say). In 1986 there was no prophylaxis.

Martinez suggested I schedule an appointment with Oncology. First, however, I should get an HIV test to confirm the AIDS diagnosis. That was a big deal in 1986. It meant going to the blood lab, where the staff practically wrapped themselves in leather and plastic when they heard the word *AIDS*. Then I walked over to Oncology and made an appointment for April 2.

After I left the hospital, I had two other things to do: Tell Mario, and tell my parents.

Mario was at work, so I called my parents. "I need to speak with both of you. I'll be there in an hour." Then I drove over to West Roxbury. Telling them was the hardest thing I'd ever done.

"Let's sit in the kitchen," I suggested. My family never sits down to talk — never — so there wasn't a right place, but I knew the kitchen would be more comfortable. I also thought back to our "coming-out" discussion in 1979 — the only time we all sat down at the kitchen table to have a family discussion.

I was twenty-nine then. Mario and I had been living

together for a year. My parents had been over to the condo —
a one-bedroom, 619-square-foot box of an apartment outside
Harvard Square. They had met Mario, but we never discussed
my sexuality, even after the tragedy of my divorce.

One summer morning, my mother called to ask for my
help installing a new sink. Manny hadn't wanted to buy it, so
he wouldn't help. I hopped on my bike and pedaled across the
river, knowing that when I got there my father wouldn't speak
to me. Coming over to help was taking sides, after all.

Barbara met me at the door and pointed me to the
bathroom, where I did the necessary tinkering. After I
finished, I sat at the kitchen table and asked her to make me
some breakfast. My reward. She put water on to boil, sat
down across from me, and delivered a line I'll never forget.

"It's a shame Mario has to sleep on the couch."

I had always told myself I would answer a direct question
about my sexuality. I wouldn't lie. I wouldn't offer information
if they didn't want to hear it, but I wouldn't pretend, either.
This qualified as a direct question.

"Oh Mom," I said, "Mario doesn't sleep on the sofa!"

"Oh no! Oh no!" she exclaimed, wringing her hands and
looking away. Then she collected herself, straightened up, and
asked, "Robert, do you go out with Jewish boys?"

"Mother," I replied, "sometimes I don't know their names,
let alone their religious affiliation!" That really undid her.

"Manny!" she shrieked, "Get in here! Your son has something to tell you!"

My father ambled into the kitchen a few moments later
and stood there, his hands in his pockets. "Yeah?" he said.

"Mario and I are boyfriends," I said.

"I know that," he replied.

Barbara turned to him, furious. "What do you mean you
know! Why didn't you tell me?"

"Oh Barbara," he groaned, waving her off, as she alter-
nately berated him and declaimed to the room how mortified
she was. My son the faegele!

"Look," said Manny, "it's fine with me what you do."

No, it's not, I thought to myself. *He just doesn't want to
have anything more said. Now or ever. In fact, thirteen years
later, their closest friends still ask if I've remarried. If it's fine,
why is Manny keeping it a secret?*

My mother picked up on his remark, however, and said, "What do you and Mario do?" My father chose that point to exit.

"What do you *mean*, what do we 'do'?" I replied, incredulous.

"Well," she struggled, "how *do* you do it?"

"How do *you* do it?" I snapped at her. "It's none of your business!"

After some back and forth, Barbara asked me to see her psychiatrist of twenty-five years, Dr. Hartwell.

"I'll see Dr. Hartwell because you're having a problem with this," I replied. "I don't have a problem. You do."

That was 1979. Now, seven years later, same kitchen table, much more serious topic. I had to "come out" again.

I pulled a chair up to the table, looked my mother in the eye, and said, "Ma, I have AIDS."

"Oh dear," she sighed, "and you just bought a new car!"

I made a mental note to process that remark later, and I waited.

"Can you give it to us?" she asked after a moment.

"No."

My father was silent. Later he asked a few questions. "What does this mean? Are you very sick?"

My mother began to weep. My father's eyes filled with tears. An acquaintance of theirs had died of AIDS the previous year. Their perception of AIDS was not pretty. They knew the stigma.

That night, I drove to Mario's apartment and told him of my diagnosis.

"What does this mean, Bob?" he asked. "Are you going to die? Does this mean I have it?" I said I didn't know. We agreed he would get tested. It turned out he was negative. That was a relief.

I also asked if he still wanted to move into the house I had just bought. "Why wouldn't I!" he said flatly. I didn't have the energy to discuss it.

Next I telephoned my brother Stephen. He was too upset to talk. His wife, Jean, called the next day, to reassure me. "I had a dream last night. The kids were teenagers and you were playing with them. I think you'll be around for a long time." *More denial,* I thought.

Over the next week, I called or visited my closest friends

with the news of my diagnosis. Linda in Florida, Kathy in New York, Steven and Bobby in Boston.

Bobby got very upset. He had been having odd problems for a number of years and was in denial himself. Night sweats, weight loss. Bobby didn't get tested for another couple years. He wasn't even out of the closet and he certainly didn't want to hear about AIDS.

A few days later, on April 2, 1986, there were two important things on my calendar: Oncology and the AIDS Action Committee.

First I went to AIDS Action, Boston's AIDS organization, to register as a client. A young man called a client advocate asked about my medical history, my financial situation, and so on. I requested medical information and asked him about volunteering. I remember very little. The word *AIDS* seemed to blot out everything else. He suggested that I look into individual psychotherapy or join a support group. I was leery of mental health professionals, however, and thought back to my mother's psychiatrist, Dr. Hartwell, whom I had met in 1979.

■

I had agreed to meet Hartwell to placate my mother, who was struggling with my sexuality. Hartwell practiced at the Veterans Administration (VA) downtown Boston facility where Barbara, who had served as a WAVE in World War II, received her care. I had never met Hartwell, although my mother had been seeing her for twenty years. Every month Hartwell mailed Barbara bags of Thorazine, lithium, and other drugs. The kitchen shelves overflowed with bottles. Hidden in our basement were shopping bags full of unused pills.

The downtown VA was an imposing, drab edifice built in the forties, replete with creaky elevators, peeling radiators, and bulging metal file cabinets.

Hartwell's lair was on the fourth floor. The door was open. She said hello to us from behind her desk, gestured towards the chairs, and lit a cigarette. Her hands trembled. Her face was lined with wrinkles.

My mother began, saying I had "devastated" her life. Mother and Hartwell traded remarks, while my mother lit a cigarette. Then Hartwell turned to me and said through the smoke, "Do you think it's right that you're doing this to your mother?"

"What am I doing to my mother?" I asked.

"Well, you're having a homosexual relationship."

"That's because I'm gay."

"Well, you're choosing to be a homosexual," Hartwell stated.

"It's not a matter of choice, Doctor!" I said.

"Yes it is," she replied firmly. "You could be heterosexual if you wanted."

"I can't be straight. I'm gay. I like *men.*"

"No," she insisted. "You could change if you wanted to!"

"Dr. Hartwell," I said, "you have to admit there are more progressive views on this matter."

She would not be deterred. "Look what you're doing to your mother!" she continued. "You *can* be straight if you want." She was relentless.

Finally I snapped. "With all due respect, Doctor, you and your colleagues here at the VA haven't been at the top of your profession for all these decades."

We wrapped the session up quickly after that! In the elevator afterwards, I told my mother, "She's a quack."

I was twenty-nine then. I'd been married and divorced in the early seventies and I knew I was gay. It was now the late seventies: Gay Liberation had happened and we gay people were doing all right. In fact, we were having quite a good time. Even the medical profession had finally acknowledged that homosexuality was not an illness. So there was no question in my mind that Hartwell was not going to "help" me.

For the next ten years, my mother and Hartwell would continue to "process" my sexuality, while smoking a small mountain of tobacco. Several months after our coming-out discussion, I had some evidence as to how well they were doing.

It was Thanksgiving Day and almost twenty family members, including half a dozen cousins and my grandmother, had gathered at my apartment for dinner. As we all sat down to dinner, my mother drawled loudly, to no one in particular, "Oh, I just don't know what to do. Both my sons are disappointments. One's a homosexual and one's a failure!"

The cousins erupted in howls and guffaws. Stevie turned to me and said, *"I'm* the failure, Robert. You're just a homosexual!" My father's sister Loretta was choking with laughter and had to leave the room.

"Why are you all laughing?" said my mother with feigned innocence, as she put her napkin in her lap. More hoots and titters. Barbara loved to start a brawl, but there were no takers this time.

■

Six years later, when my client advocate at AIDS Action suggested therapy to me, these were some of the memories I had. Although dubious about individual therapy and psychiatrists in particular, I was desperate enough to agree to look into support groups.

After meeting with the Advocate, I drove to the hospital in a fog. By the time I got to Oncology, I had myself a little more together. The waiting room was large and quiet. There were about a dozen women seated. I was the only man. *Breast cancer,* I thought. The staff spoke in hushed tones. One woman was weeping. It was a sad place.

The staff were well trained, sympathetic, and understanding. They knew how to talk with terminally ill people. They knew you could get crazy. One nurse I really liked was Jane. She was smart. Smarter than the doctors. I had some good talks with her about efficacy and dosage. Ultimately I talked her into buying a house.

A receptionist showed me into an office. After a couple minutes, a large masked figure walked in and sat down. He was young, blond, and beefy. He was also reserved and virtually antiseptic. Let's call him Mr. Clean.

"So you have Kaposi's sarcoma," he began, flipping through my records. "Let me tell you a little about it and how we treat it."

"Fine," I said.

"The spots you have are called lesions. Let's take a look."

I rolled up my pant leg. He put on rubber gloves and pressed his thumb to one spot, then the other. Then he took a sheet of white paper and drew what looked like the Pillsbury Doughboy, a crude Pillsbury Doughboy with only one foot. On the figure's left ankle, Mr. Clean marked a little black spot. Then he filed the drawing in my record as baseline documentation.

Here's what it looked like:

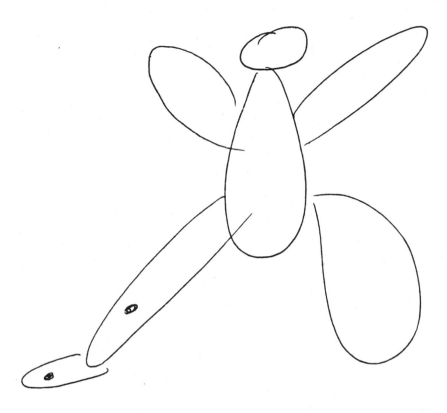

"How long do I have to live, Doctor?" I asked.

"I don't have that information," Clean replied.

This is a Harvard teaching hospital, I thought. *There are piles and piles of information around here! What does he mean, we don't have that information?*

"What do the statistics show?"

He sidestepped my question, saying, "I don't really need that level of detail in order to treat you."

"This information is important to *me,* Doctor," I explained. "I have lots of decisions to make, and not just about medical treatment. There's my job, my IRA, insurance — not to mention my estate. I need to know how long I'm going to live."

I wanted to be active and practical. If I could expect to live six years, I would increase my disability insurance. If I had only six months, I would increase my life insurance and quit my job immediately. I also wanted to evaluate treatment options in the light of my life span. If a treatment would make me sick for six months and I only had nine months to live, I wouldn't consider it. But if I had five years, then I would.

"We're going to treat you with Velban," he said. "Do the best we can. Probabilities about how long you're going to live don't really affect the course of treatment."

"How does chemo work with people with KS?" I responded. "Does it ever do more harm than good?" I grilled him about dosage and efficacy and side effects. He knew little. He was new to the hospital and young — and seemed startled by a patient who asked questions.

"How do you know how much to give me?" I asked. It turned out they gave everyone the same dosage of Velban. No options. This is what we do. Period.

This did not set well with me.

Dosage is something to watch carefully. I've always known that. When I was a kid, Mother took a megatranquilizer called Thorazine. Manny used to nag her to take her meds. Barbara didn't want to be overly tranquilized, so she didn't always take as much as Manny wanted her to, but she took a lot. Just how much I didn't realize, until I was sixteen.

It was 1966 and I had discovered marijuana. My friends were talking about various fun pills, so my thoughts turned to Thorazine. Mother took eight huge 100-mg pills a day. After school one afternoon, I took *one* pill ... and slept for two days. Right through school. I got up occasionally to use the bathroom. My parents didn't notice anything. That's when it occurred to me that Mother was taking too much medication.

Naturally, when Dr. Clean began describing Velban to me, I wanted to discuss dosage!

"Doctor, I'm little — just five-feet-four — and I weigh a hundred-twenty. It doesn't make sense to give me the same dose as a six-foot man. This stuff is poison, after all!"

"We don't adjust dosage for body weight," he responded smoothly. "It doesn't work that way."

"Oh. Well, what do you adjust it for?"

For other cancers, I knew the oncologists set chemotherapy dosage according to the nature of the cancer, how fast it was spreading, and where it was located. Barbara had had breast cancer and I'd been through this secondhand. I'd heard about combining chemotherapies and checking white blood cell counts.

For the dosage decision to be so cut-and-dried, something had to be very wrong. Either the procedure was nonsensical or Clean was following it blindly.

How am I going to get information out of this guy? I thought to myself. I decided to try another approach.

"How long will we do it for?"

"That depends on how well you respond."

"How will we know when to stop?"

"We really have to take it step by step."

"What's a step?"

"Well, we'll have to see if and when you start to respond."

"How will you know when I'm responding?"

"The KS will stop spreading."

"Will we stop the chemotherapy then?"

"Perhaps."

I decided to change tack. "What is the probability that I'll have a complete response? Or a partial response? For that matter, what's the probability I won't have any response?"

"For the individual patient it doesn't make any difference what the numbers are," Clean replied. He didn't know how to say, "I don't know."

"What are the side effects?" I asked. "When should I expect them? Am I going to lose my hair?"

"Maybe."

"What can I do to minimize or deal with side effects?"

He promised to get that information.

Well, that's something, I said to myself.

I returned again to the issue of prognosis. "How long do I have to live?"

I insisted. Finally Clean said, "Well, if you must have a number, I'd say about a year."

"Okay, I can deal with that, but please show me the data. I want to see why you think so. Can you get me written information on people with KS?"

"I don't think we have that here at BI."

"Then where do we go to get it?"

"I'm afraid I can't answer that question."

Here we go again! I thought.

So far, the meeting had been very frustrating. The prognosis ("You have about a year") wasn't backed up with any logic or data I could understand. I didn't know what to make of anything Dr. Clean said. Maybe his proposed course of action was reasonable, maybe not. I couldn't tell. His opinions were useless to me without further information.

This first meeting with Dr. Clean had lasted longer than he'd expected. He had other patients scheduled and I'd taken more than my twenty minutes. Nonetheless, I came away unsatisfied. I decided to call my cousin Dana, who was a doctor in Omaha, and ask him for information on AIDS, KS, and chemotherapy.

In retrospect, I think Clean would have been more sympathetic if I'd been a man with prostate cancer or a woman with breast cancer. He might have sought the information I requested and treated my condition more aggressively. Today I would ask him how many PWAs with KS he'd treated and how many articles he'd read on the subject.

I've learned a lot since then. In general, I assume the information that medical staff give me is incomplete. They have to show me that they're up-to-date. I make them explain their logic and you should, too. Every time something doesn't make sense, say, "It doesn't make sense!" Explain where you think you hear a gap or a contradiction in their logic.

Even if your doctor's information is up-to-date, it's based on studies conducted eighteen months ago. What treatments were given, how they worked, who responded. I always look ahead to what HIV will be like in two or three years. The doctors look backwards.

April 9. Frightened, I reported for my first chemotherapy treatment. Dr. Clean had run some of my questions by the head of the Oncology Department, Glenn Bubbley, whom I decided to refer to as Bubbles. Same answers. Bubbles was too busy to deal with me at that point, but we ultimately saw each other a lot. I began the treatment.

A few days later, I drove down to Manhattan to visit my friend Kathy. It was a difficult visit. The lesion on my foot was becoming painful. I had trouble walking. The prospect of losing my mobility was a nightmare.

Kathy knew people with AIDS and was distraught. In a lighter moment, I remember her saying, "Aren't you going to be pissed off at yourself if you're alive and healthy five years from now and you wasted these years? Don't pine away and wait to die. Live a little. Go to Provincetown. Have a cocktail!" In retrospect, it was the best advice I received.

When I returned to Boston, a packet had arrived from Dr. Dana in Omaha, with three articles about AIDS and Kaposi's sarcoma. I studied them carefully. One article contained graphs showing the percent of AIDS patients alive over time. According to one graph, 30 percent of people with AIDS were still living after three years. Then the graph flattened out because they lacked data. It looked something like this:

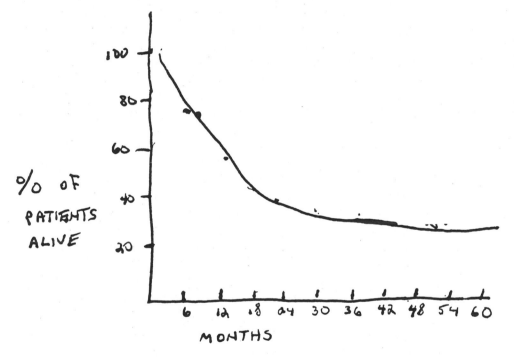

Also, I found a statement that PWAs with KS and no other symptoms lived longer than those who had additional symptoms. This was the first hopeful information I received.

People with KS and no other symptoms, I thought. *That's me! People who are less sick!* I read and reread the article. *How long did PWAs with KS and no other symptoms live in this study?* I wondered. The authors did not say.

If I get through one year, I'm off that steep slope, I

thought. *The first year's the most dangerous. If I get to three years, things flatten out...*

Excited, I telephoned Dana with questions. He couldn't help. No one had yet been diagnosed with AIDS in Omaha. He had no experience and no one to talk to.

April 16. My second chemotherapy appointment. I brought the articles with me and handed them to Dr. Clean as I sat down.

"What is this?" asked Clean.

"Information about KS survival rates. I think we should discuss it."

He scanned the material quickly. *Too quickly,* I thought.

"Doesn't this show I'm likely to be alive in three years?" I queried.

Clean glanced at the graphs again. "Maybe it could be interpreted that way. But there are so many variables!" He shook his head and continued, "You must understand that this information doesn't change how I'm going to treat you. It's sort of academic, really."

"It will change how I *let* you treat me, Doctor," I said evenly. "If I have three years to live, that's very different from nine months. For one thing, I'll keep working for a while. I won't want treatments to make me too sick to work. Furthermore," I continued, "if I might be alive in three to five years, maybe they'll develop some treatment in the meantime. Maybe you should just keep this KS under control. Give me less chemotherapy, perhaps. How much chemo does it take to wipe out the KS, as opposed to slowing it down? If wiping it out means taking a lot more poison, I might not be interested."

I pointed to a portion of a second article, concerning a different population afflicted with KS: kidney transplant patients who were receiving immunosuppressive drugs. These drugs prevent rejection of a donated organ by disabling the body's response to foreign substances. When the kidney patients stopped taking immunosuppressive drugs, their KS cleared up! It looked as if the body's normal immune system could handle KS just fine.

From this I reasoned: *The weakening of my immune system by HIV is the problem. KS is the symptom. If we could treat HIV directly, my body would handle KS on its own. We should find a way to treat the HIV itself.*

I presented this logic to Dr. Clean. He was distressed.

"But you have KS! We're treating the KS."

"I understand that," I replied, "and that's better than nothing. But I would rather be treating the underlying *cause* of my KS."

"We have no treatment for HIV!"

"But you might in two years!" I insisted. *His logic is bad,* I said to myself. *He's not really thinking; he's just following procedures.*

But I'd learned enough to form a working hypothesis: I could count on living three years. And during those three years, a treatment would probably be developed that would slow down the HIV virus itself. So I figured I might have three to five years, perhaps closer to five.

(If I were learning I was HIV-positive today, my working hypothesis would be different. I might reason that an effective treatment would be developed within the next three years — something like insulin, for diabetes. Therefore, my task would be to stay as healthy as I could until treatment arrived. I would also assume this new treatment would keep me going until an even more effective treatment was found five or ten years later. Optimistic working hypotheses work well for me.)

This rationale gave me a glimmer of hope. It also motivated me to make decisions: First, I would keep working. Second, I would refinance the house, once Mario and I had moved in, and get Mario's name on the deed. That way, if I died, the house would automatically pass to Mario, outside of the will — and the bank could not call in the mortgage. Finally, I would think about finding a support group.

Two days later, I returned to Yankee. First I stopped by the personnel office and talked to Terry. He was very understanding. He explained how Yankee's disability insurances worked. When I got too sick to work, I would receive 60 percent of my salary.

"In the meantime, do whatever you have to do to take care of yourself. Doctor appointments and so forth. We've already spoken with Mercedes."

Mercedes met with me next. She was very supportive. In my absence, she had reassigned my staff to other managers and found some low-priority projects I could work on. Busy-work, really.

The company was trying to do the right thing. In contrast, New England Telephone was firing people with AIDS at that very moment.

The chemotherapy seemed to work. A couple of new lesions popped out, then no more. But maybe chemo made it worse — I didn't start limping till after I started chemo. The side effects were slight: constipation and slight hair loss. Fevers, too, which Clean and Bubbles both mistakenly attributed to HIV. That really disturbed me. Now we know the fevers were a side effect of chemo.

Dr. Clean never said exactly how many treatments it would be. In fact, we continued for ten weeks. Finally, in late June I said, "When are we going to stop this?" He thought we should "play it by ear."

"What does that mean?" I asked.

"Keep on with these doses," he said.

"Well, let's cut back or stop or something," I said.

I saw no benefit in continuing. We had met my objective — to stabilize the situation. It was time to think of next steps. Clean was doubtful, but I insisted. We agreed he would monitor me once a month.

■

Over the summer, the shock of my diagnosis wore off somewhat and the stress of moving subsided. I successfully refinanced the house. Dr. Martinez left Beth Israel in July. His departure surprised and disappointed me. When I inquired, I learned that he had been a resident — like most doctors at Health Care Associates, the clinic I went to at BI. Residents stay only a year before moving on. I didn't bother to request a new primary care physician, because I was seeing Dr. Clean regularly. As for Clean himself, I wasn't thrilled with him, but he seemed adequate. I didn't believe I could get anyone better.

In September, I enrolled in a weekly support group for PWAs, run by a clinical social worker. By the third meeting, I was dissatisfied. I wanted to focus on living, but the other participants talked mostly about illness, side effects, and planning funerals, even though they were no sicker than I. I never heard about friends, family, or work.

Attendance was worse than irregular. People went once or

twice and then never again. Each new arrival described the shock of getting diagnosed — and ruminated on his impending death.

At the fourth session, I turned to the facilitator and said, "There's no continuity here. It's disruptive to always be starting anew, listening to the diagnosis story and so on."

"Why is that a problem?"

"Because I'd like to get to know people. Get beyond what's wrong with them physically. If we had some continuity, maybe we'd get some real support. As it is, people come once, blurt out their stories, and leave."

"Why don't you deal with that in group?" she replied.

Don't therapize me, I thought. *This isn't about my psyche. It's about how you set expectations with group members.*

"Maybe you should tell newcomers they must come regularly before you admit them to the group. If you set expectations first, we could deal with whatever comes up later in group."

She was silent.

I thought of Hartwell and groaned. I stopped going after that. It would be a couple years before I tried a support group again.

■

I've explained why I question dosages. My parents actually trained me to question everything, starting with their sanity.

My mother had a lot of experience with the mental health system and with hospitals. Over the years, she was in and out of institutions. I often got ambiguous or contradictory information. When that happens, you need to gather additional information, make a judgment, and act. Don't get stuck.

Even as a little boy, I knew to use my own judgment. I knew when mother needed to go into the hospital and I knew when she was ready to come out. Often, she was ready to come out but my father wasn't ready to have her home. It would mean some work and some adjustment, which he found difficult. If the doctor said, "No, she's not ready to come out," and I knew she *was* ready, then I knew the doctor was wrong. Even as a child. I was being trained to deal with conflicting information and ambiguous situations.

Someone had to supervise my mother's care: what medications she took, how much, how frequently, and how long the doctors kept her in the hospital. My father couldn't supervise. He never voiced an opinion. He let the doctors decide when to put her in the hospital and when to let her out. "I'll do what the doctors say. They know what they're doing." Consequently, I became the supervisor and dealt with the ambiguity.

Ambiguous information is stressful. We want to get away from it. But sticking your head in the ground does not change reality; you only give away control. Unfortunately, there is no simple recipe for coping with ambiguity. No prearranged Things To Do list to follow. But there are things you can do, every step of the way.

In this book I'll describe the strategies I've developed for managing ambiguity and working the system. I had some of these coping skills *before* HIV and gained others after. I'll tell you right now: If I had blindly followed the advice of my doctors — if I hadn't questioned them vigorously — I'd be dead.

There are several basic skills everyone with HIV needs. The first step is recognizing that life with HIV is ambiguous at best. After that, you'll find yourself much further ahead if you can:

- Set your own objectives
- Gather information
- Solve problems creatively
- Negotiate
- Pay attention to details
- Stay motivated

You don't need to excel at every task. When you have trouble, seek help. Get friends to do it with you. Or for you. Or have them show you how.

Let's consider *your* life experiences for a moment. Have you already managed situations that are relevant to the HIV bureaucracy? I'll bet you have. We all have valuable and unrecognized coping skills. Have you ever spotted a contradiction or a loophole? Questioned authority? These are skills used in managing HIV.

Let's use the following quiz to assess your untapped skills...

HOW EQUIPPED ARE YOU TO COPE WITH AMBIGUITY?
Rate yourself on each item below, then total the points.

Add one point if...

____ One of your parents is mentally ill

____ One of your parents is an alcoholic

____ You are in a recovery program

____ You have successfully filed an auto insurance claim and collected

____ You have traveled abroad

____ You knew in 1984 that Vanessa Williams would become a star

Add two points if you have ever...

____ Been mistreated by a doctor before HIV — or know someone who was

____ Been "treated" by a psychiatrist for homosexuality

____ Taught kindergarten

____ Bought a house

____ Gotten a divorce

____ Come out

____ Worked your way through college by selling marijuana

Subtract two points if you...

____ Went to parochial school

____ Are still Catholic

____ Still live with your parents

____ Believe it's your fault you got HIV

____ Believe insurance companies are altruistic

____ Believe almost all doctors are competent

____ Think American cars are just as good as Japanese cars

____ Have never heard of John Waters

____ **TOTAL**

RATING

11–20: You already have the skills necessary to handle HIV. You wasted your money buying this book.

5–10: You have a B.S. in "Life Experiences!" When you complete this book, you will have a graduate degree in Living with HIV.

0–4: Wake up or *They Will Kill You!*

Below 0: Are you sure you want to read this book? If so, get a friend to read it with you or to you.

■

HIV, like any life-threatening disease, can be overwhelming. You struggle to keep a sense of perspective. In the process, you may question old assumptions. How long will I live? What do I want out of life? *What's important to me?* Your priorities and values may change significantly.

Partners can help you deal with these issues. Depending on your needs, they can provide emotional support, help figure out ambiguous information, keep track of bills and other details, or bang on desks for you. The critical thing is: Partners can help keep the system focused on what's important to you.

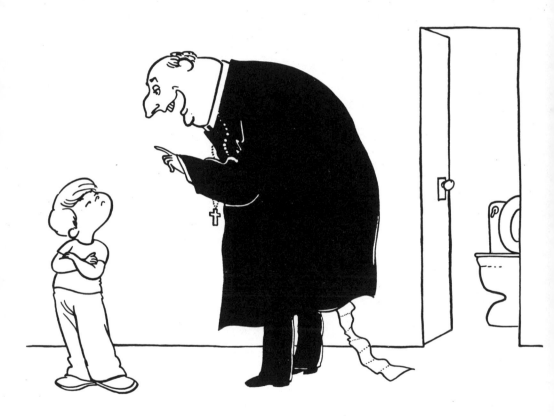

MORAL: **Question Authority.**
Living with HIV is ambiguous.
Even the experts will often be wrong.

COPING WITH AMBIGUITY
Use this worksheet to see how these concepts might apply to you.

1. When have I come out before? What about?

2. Do I have more information on some HIV topics than my doctor does? Which topics?

3. What do I need to know more about right now?

4. Whom can I ask or what can I do to get this information?

5. What are my working hypotheses at this moment?

    I think a real treatment for HIV might be available in 199___ .

    I think a cure might be discovered by _____ .

    I expect to live at least _____ years because

    _____ .

    In order to stay alive until _____ , I need to

    _____

    _____

    _____

6. What's important to me:

    _____

    _____

7. Who can I talk this over with?

2

Working the System

Y ou can't buy an ice cream cone in America without encountering a system.

Now you have HIV — or someone you know does. A new and bewildering landscape will shortly come into view. It includes medical facilities, insurance companies, your employer's personnel department, government programs, and AIDS agencies. A world of organizations, acronyms, and forms. It may seem as if you have entered the Twilight Zone. It's the HIV system.

The good news is: You've been working systems all your life. You have more skills than you think. *You don't need to fear the HIV bureaucracy.* Instead, get to know the system — and work it!

Here are some of the questions you're probably thinking about:

- Who knows — or can find out — if I test positive?
- Which should I deal with first — my medical situation or my financial situation?
- How do I get insurance? (health, disability, life)
- Who knows or can find out if I seek treatment?
- How do I get medical treatment if I don't have insurance?
- What if the system already knows I'm HIV-positive?
- Should I just let my doctor tell me what to do?
- What kinds of information do I need to make decisions?

In this chapter I'll show you how, with a little information, imagination, and system-sense, you can get inside bureaucracies and make them work for you.

THE MEDICAL SYSTEM: KNOW HOW IT WORKS

What would happen if you arranged to fly from New York to L.A. without understanding the air travel system? You'd pay the standard price — perhaps $1000 instead of $400. You'd check your baggage. And they'd lose it.

Medical care is like air travel. If you know the system, you get more for your money. You get better service. This chapter outlines the basic principles of working the medical system and other parts of the HIV bureaucracy.

The first step is: *Watch the moving parts.*

Let's consider a real-life example of a system: Burger King. "We do it *your* way!" the ad says. If you always order a regular Whopper, you probably get what you ask for. You've never had reason to question the system.

But what if you don't want that suspicious-looking sauce? What happens if you place a special order? Has your Whopper ever come out *not* the way you ordered? Where do you think the mistake happened? Think of all the moving parts. Was it...

- What you said to the cashier?
- What the cashier thought he heard?
- What he punched into the terminal?
- What popped out on the screen in the kitchen?
- The cook who did not read the screen correctly?
- Someone who put ketchup in the mustard container?
- Someone who put the wrong hamburger on your tray?
- That your original cashier picked up the wrong tray?
- That you picked up the wrong tray?

See all the parts? Each of them is a potential source of error.

System Law #1:
> *Systems have moving parts.*
> *The more parts, the more errors.*

Have you ever noticed how no one takes responsibility for the whole process? And how no one admits to making a mistake?

As a customer, you can, of course, take steps to prevent mistakes — for example, have the cashier read back your order to you. Even so, there will be some mistakes. So you act to correct them after the fact. You send the Whopper back.

Sometimes, however, mistakes work in your favor. For example, you may get two Whoppers instead of one. Just because systems are complex doesn't mean you always lose. Not at all. Some errors will be in your favor.

Before looking at the HIV bureaucracy, think back to when you encountered other systems:

- Getting a driver's license
- Booking a ticket on an airline
- Applying for a loan
- Interviewing for a job
- Paying your taxes
- Getting reimbursed by your health insurance company.

Pick a system you mastered. Think of all the moving parts.

- Who did you speak to first?
- Who eventually helped you?
- If you submitted written information, where did it go?
- Were there foul-ups or mistakes?
- Did you find a way to make the system work faster or better?
- If not, do you know someone who did?

Watching the moving parts will help you get better service from all sorts of HIV systems. Let's start with your medical facility.

Getting medical care means dealing with a bureaucracy. It's not you and the doctor sitting in a quiet little room with a stethoscope and a black bag. Open the door and take a look. You and your doctor are a little part of a bigger system!

Consider the parallels between air travel and medical care, for a moment.

Traditional thinking has your primary care physician as the pilot, while the copilot is the oncologist or another specialist — perhaps a radiation therapist or opthamologist. You, the patient, are back in the economy section. Your job is to sit still until it's all over. Of course, if you're clever you may have found a way to get into first class and get a free drink!

The nurses function as flight attendants. They try to make you comfortable. What does that mean? Sometimes it means dealing with your side effects, which is quite tricky. The nurse knows side effects because he'll have to deal with them, not the doctor. He is the one who thinks to say, "I'll get you some saltines or ginger ale because you're going to get nauseated after this treatment."

In this and other ways, the nurses are more important than flight attendants, although those of you who really need the pillow and the extra drink may not agree.

Meanwhile, up in the cockpit, the pilot is responsible for coordinating the critical aspects of air travel. He gets you from point A to point B without crashing. In the traditional view, that is the doctor's role.

A progressive primary care physician might suggest that you're the copilot. He is in charge, but you have real "input."

As I see it, however, *you* are the pilot and the doctor is the copilot. The pilot is there to help *you*. You set the destination, coordinate the gathering and review of vital information, and make the major decisions. In reality, few primary care physicians do all these things and even fewer patients do. But I'm getting ahead of myself. Back to the traditional view, where you're sitting in economy class, chatting with the nurse.

Now consider the medical facility itself. It parallels the airline. The airline chooses services to deliver — various routes and flight schedules. It organizes the staff and machines to deliver service, and it has policies for maintaining and repairing the planes. Finally, it monitors some of the results, like the percentage of flights on time and the number of crashes.

The hospital decides what services to offer (whether to have CAT scans, for example) and sets service standards like how many hours it is willing to have people wait in the Emergency Room, not unlike the airline's on-time arrival goals.

Both airlines and hospitals use detailed procedures for hiring staff and monitoring their performance. The airline sets standards for pilots — how many hours of previous flight time they must have, what kind of experience, how many hours they may fly before they must rest, how much alcohol they can have in their blood when they take off, and so forth. Similarly, the hospital sets standards for physicians based on their skill levels and previous experience, and it monitors patient caseload and the number of hours the staff work.

These internal procedures are invisible to consumers, but service quality is not. People choose not to use certain airlines based on factors like how often the flights are late, how frequently baggage is lost, the number of DC-10s in the fleet, and whether engines have recently fallen off the planes. *Some airlines are better than others.*

Similarly, some hospitals are better than others. Some hospitals have strict guidelines about how well they treat people with HIV, just like some airlines define a family as a married man and woman and their children, while others will define a family as two people living together, irrespective of gender.

The hospital blood lab is a lot like the airline's baggage handling system. It's not the glamorous, high-tech part of the system, but it critically affects the quality of service. And it's often the weak point. You probably know the basics of the baggage handling system, in particular, that a passenger may carry on two pieces of luggage. Many of you probably stand on your head to get everything into two bags. If it won't all fit, you put the important stuff in your carry-on bags and check the unimportant luggage.

Why do you do this?

Because you know how baggage handling works. The system has a thousand moving parts, little accountability, and abundant opportunities for error. Luggage can be mislabeled, the label can be misread or ignored, the label can fall off, the luggage itself can fall off the conveyor. And so on.

As a passenger, you try to minimize errors by checking to see that your luggage is properly labeled. As a hospital patient, have you ever thought to glance to see if the phlebotomist has labeled your blood correctly? Or labeled it at all?

Similarly, when you have a close connection to make, you know there's likely to be a problem with baggage, so you take precautions. Have you ever thought about not having your blood drawn at 4:30 p.m., especially on a Friday? It may get misplaced and sit overnight on a radiator. Then they tell you "it got lost."

Recently, Beth Israel lost my friend Rachel's blood — ten tubes of it. When they called her, they said, "Hi. We're terribly sorry, but we lost your blood. Could you come in again?"

"What do you think they meant by 'lost'?" she giggled as she recounted the call.

Well, think of all the moving parts. Did the lab...

- Put the blood in the correct vials?

- Label the vials correctly?
- Get the vials to the lab without breaking them?
- Perform the correct tests?
- Analyze the results properly?
- Record the results?
- Enter the results into the computer correctly and under the right name?

Who knows?

Do you think this is an isolated problem? Read on.

One day I sat in the lab waiting room. It was hot and crowded and I was groggy. The attendant, a young man named Julio, picked up a test tube and lab slip and muttered, "Reemer! Mrs. Reemer." No one moved. He had a strong accent and did not enunciate clearly. I stared dully at the magazine in my lap. "Reemer!" he repeated again. My name is Robert Rimer. RYE-MER.

The eighty-year-old woman across from me slowly got to her feet and shuffled across the room. Julio sat her down and began to draw blood. Suddenly I realized what was happening. He was putting her blood in a test tube with *my* labels on it. Pretty soon, the doctor would be telling me that my hysterectomy had been a success. And someone else was going to get some bad news and pointed questions about their sex life.

I stood up and said, "Excuse me. You've made a mistake. You've got the wrong person."

Julio beamed. "Thank you, sir! You next!" Smiling and nodding, he fixed the label with my name to her blood.

"Did you see what he did!" I said to the whole room, in a loud voice. "He's putting her blood in my test tube!"

Nurses gathered at the door. One pointed. Two of them tittered. The first to regain her composure put on a businesslike expression and walked up to me.

"What seems to be the matter?"

"That man is mislabeling the blood samples!"

"Oh, I see." She walked over to Julio, spoke a few quiet words, got the labels rearranged, and redirected Julio to the next task.

This was not the last time I had problems with the blood lab. They've lost blood repeatedly. Nor was it my sole encounter with Julio. We've had other run-ins since then. In fact, Julio is notorious. Years later, I spoke to a hospital supervisor about a scheduling snafu in a different department. As we chatted he confided, "If you think things are screwed up here, you should hear the complaints we get about the blood lab!"

The point is: *Systems have lots of Julios — and people who are new on the job or tired or unaware of changes in procedures.* It's up to you to watch out for them. While you're watching, keep in mind that errors can also be opportunities. As my mother taught me long ago, some of the system's errors will be in your favor.

Barbara knew about systems inside and outside the hospital. She once burned clothes in the dryer — left them in a couple hours on high heat, I guess. I found them when they started to smoke.

I didn't think anything of it. Housework was not Mother's forte. "Too bad you burned your clothes!" I said.

"Oh," she chirped as she dropped the clothes in the wastebasket, "I'll file a claim with the insurance company!"

"Gee, Mom," I asked, "do you think this is covered by our homeowner's policy?"

"It doesn't make any difference if it's covered, Robert," she explained. "What counts is whether they pay you!" I raised my eyebrows quizzically. She continued, "If you put in the claim, they might pay you. If you don't put in the claim, they certainly won't pay you. So let's just do it and see what happens!"

To my surprise, the company paid the claim. Barbara understood how the system worked. She applied system-sense to her problem and got a new wardrobe!

Working a system calls for applying a mix of information, imagination, and system-sense to a problem. Consider a more common example: airline overbooking. We all know the airlines overbook. What happens if you get bumped? The airline puts you on the next flight and gives you a free ticket. That's how the system works.

What would happen if your budget was really tight and you wanted a free ticket? Could you arrange to get bumped? What if you chose to arrive fifteen minutes before flight time on Thanksgiving?

In the next section, I'll describe how you can make errors in the blood lab work to your advantage. The rule is: Sometimes you take preventive measures to make sure there are no

2. Working the System

errors. Other times you just let the system work the way it does.

TESTING: FIRST ENCOUNTERS WITH THE HIV SYSTEM

When you find out you're HIV-positive, you must deal with at least two systems: the medical facility and the insurance companies. You need to:

- assess your medical situation;
- get group health insurance, if you don't have it; and
- get group disability income insurance, if you don't have it.

The problem is, if you treat your medical situation first, you may be prevented from getting appropriate health and disability coverage later. I was fortunate enough to have these things lined up. But I've helped dozens of people since then who were not so fortunate.

It's common practice to take your HIV test anonymously. There are certain people who you don't want knowing your HIV status: insurance companies, employers, landlords, etc. They don't need the information to give you good service. In fact, they'll use it against you if they get it.

The problem is much bigger than keeping your HIV status off the record. And much more complicated.

It is risky to get *any* HIV-related tests, treatments, or diagnoses done under your own name, until you have a group health insurance policy and a disability income insurance policy. In fact, it's risky to get any tests that indicate a condition which would lead a normal person to take an HIV test.

T4 TESTING

If your doctor knows you've tested HIV-positive, she'll think, "Oh my God, you're gonna get sick. We gotta run tests to see what action is required right now."

What do you do? Your doctor wants to deal promptly with your medical issues. Your T4 cell count, in particular, will show if you're at immediate risk for infections. Of course, your situation may not be critical at all. Even if you appear perfectly healthy, however, you should get a T4 test.

But, you should get T4 information anonymously, for the same reason you got your HIV status anonymously. Unfortunately, there are few anonymous T4 test sites today. If you can't find one, you must work the existing system.

Here are two scenarios depicting how you might get your T4 count anonymously. They may not be the best ways. My intent is to encourage you to create and explore options.

The direct route...

Ask your doctor hypothetical questions.

"Doctor, if I ask you a hypothetical question, do you have to put it in my medical record? I don't want hypothetical discussions in my record...

"If I tested HIV-positive and wanted to get my T4 level tested anonymously, would there be some way you could arrange that? Is there somewhere you could send me? Would you be upset if I went somewhere else and used someone else's name?

"Also, Doctor, what other tests would you do if I tested HIV-positive? Would you give me any prophylaxis?"

And so on.

Your doctor might be able to work something out with you. After all, she knows the system better than you do!

The indirect route...

Remember the discussion about blood labs in the previous section? T4 testing is a time when errors can be opportunities. You could find a friend who has been HIV-positive for a while and is scheduled for blood tests. What would happen if you took your friend's blood slips and medical card over to the blood lab?

Your friend would get your results a week later. If your T4 count was quite different from his most recent results, the scene might go something like this:

"Oh, Alphonse!" exclaims the doctor, "your T4 count went up 200 points! Isn't that amazing!"

"Could I see that number?" replies Alphonse. "That's wonderful, but it must be a mistake. You know how they are in the lab! Let's do it over."

And they would. Meanwhile, Alphonse gives you your results — and still gets his own correct reading a week later.

It's almost foolproof. Even if the lab tech somehow remembered Alphonse's face and asked why you had the wrong lab papers and hospital card, you could say, "I must have picked the wrong papers off the desk! I'm sorry! I'll go get the right slips." Then you scurry out of the room.

That's one way to get your T4 results anonymously. Use your imagination. Be creative. Hospitals never ask for picture IDs.

Remember Rachel, who told me about the ten test tubes of lost blood? She got really creative and made up a new name (something like Tawdry LaFrance) and found a new doctor. The doctor does all her HIV-related tests under that name. Since "Tawdry" is a fictitious person and has no insurance policy, Rachel pays cash for those tests. Everything else is done under her real name and billed to the insurance company.

As I said before, the T4 test indicates how much your immune system has been damaged and whether you need to begin medical treatment. Basically, *the T4 test tells you whether medical stuff is more important than financial stuff right now.*

Many people assume that medical issues are more important than financial. On the other hand, even people with low T4 counts sometimes feel that financial matters are more important, particularly if they need to line up disability insurance or group health insurance. Here's how you decide.

Assuming your T4s are above 500, antivirals can wait a few months while you work out insurance issues. Usually there's no reason to begin other HIV-related prophylaxes immediately. Of course, you should be getting flu shots and other preventive medicine. Your priority should be financial prophylaxis, which I'll discuss in the next section.

If your T4s are below 400 or 500, most doctors will start treatment. If you don't have both health insurance and disability insurance, try to keep HIV treatments off your medical record until you do. Options include: having a friend ask her doctor about treatments for you, going with your lover or best friend to his doctor, or speaking to your doctor off the record.

Let's assume your T4 level is 400. What would your doctor do?

- Give you a pneumonia shot?
- Give you a flu shot?
- Test you for tuberculosis?
- Prescribe an antiviral?

The pneumonia and flu shots are easy to arrange. You could ask a doctor if that's what he would (hypothetically) prescribe and then make arrangements to get them elsewhere. Similarly, concerning the antiviral, you could ask, "If I had a friend who were HIV-positive and his T4 count were such and such, what antiviral would you recommend? And what dosage?"

If hypothetical discussions seem unworkable or you don't have a doctor, there are at least four other ways to choose an antiviral:

1) Go with an HIV-infected friend to her doctor.

2) Call the Gay Men's Health Crisis (GMHC) Treatment Line in New York. They'll tell you exactly what to do. They'll say it's information, not advice, but you can put it all together.

3) Call Project Inform in San Francisco.

4) Call your local AIDS service organization (ASO) or ACT-UP chapter. They may have more up-to-date information than your doctor.

■

Once you've decided upon an antiviral, you can buy it through other sources for a few months, if your doctor can't get it for you without putting it in your medical record. Your options include:

1) Buyers clubs. These drug distribution organizations advertise in the National Association of People with AIDS (NAPWA) newsletter, various HIV-positive publications, and gay newspapers.

2) HIV-positive friends may have some extra pills or know someone who does.

3) AIDS service organizations sometimes discreetly give out antivirals. You may not have to register as a client.

4) Take out a personal ad in an AIDS organization newsletter, "Looking for XYZ antiviral."

Now let's discuss more fully why you want to keep information off the record.

DEFENSIVE DRIVING IN THE HIV SYSTEM: GETTING GROUP HEALTH INSURANCE

Your doctor is concerned with treating you medically. She does not think about your financial situation — but you had better do so, before it's too late.

Unless your job provides group health and disability insurance, your financial situation may be shaky.

You may have group health insurance through your employer right now. Does that mean you're all set? What if you get laid off? Or want to leave your job? Can you take your health insurance with you? What happens if you switch jobs?

Even ethical, compassionate employers have incentives to discriminate against HIV-positive people. Therefore, you must take care that your HIV status is not widely known.

You certainly don't want to tell a prospective employer that you're HIV-infected. Sometimes an employer's payments for group insurance are based on the number of claims filed. A job applicant with HIV looks like a very expensive employee! Obviously you should not draw attention to yourself by cross-examining a potential employer about health benefits. But successful candidates are typically given an opportunity to speak with a benefits person before accepting a job offer. After all, benefits are part of your compensation. Here are some questions you should ask about health and disability insurance:

- How much will the policy cost me?
- Will I have to fill out an application?
- Will I be subject to medical screening?
- Will I have to authorize release of my medical records?
- Is there a waiting period before the policy is in effect?
- Is there a pre-existing condition clause?
- If so, what is the exclusionary period? How long will the insurance company deny coverage for a pre-existing condition?
- May I see any doctor I wish or must I pick from a list of affiliated doctors?
- When I change jobs or leave the company, can I convert from a group to an individual policy? If so...
- What would an individual policy cost?
- Will the policy cover prescription medications?
- Can I keep the policy indefinitely?
- What is the lifetime cap, once I convert to individual coverage?

Here's a comparison of typical group and individual insurances. As you can see, group policies are preferable.

	GROUP HEALTH or DISABILITY	INDIVIDUAL HEALTH or DISABILITY
COST	Less	More
APPLICATION REQUIRED?	No	Yes
MEDICAL SCREENING	Rarely	Sometimes
MEDICAL RECORDS	Rarely	Yes
WAITING PERIOD	0–3 months	0–3 months
PRE-EXISTING CONDITION EXCLUSIONARY PERIOD	0–24 months	Life of policy -or- 12–24 months
SCOPE OF COVERAGE	More extensive	Less extensive

When filling out a job application you are dealing with a system. What if the application asks about HIV? If you're unemployed or your current job is so unacceptable that you have to leave, you may have to omit references to previous HIV-related illnesses in order to take care of yourself.

The rule is:

Be careful what you tell the system.

When people change jobs, they often change insurance carriers, too. For HIV-positive people, this transition can be risky, because the insurance companies use what is called a "pre-existing condition clause" to limit their costs. Among other things, the pre-existing condition clause was designed to prevent pregnant women from seeking a job so that their maternity costs would be paid for by the insurance carrier.

During the pre-existing condition exclusionary period, the new carrier can decline to cover HIV-related illnesses. Consider continuing your old insurance (at your expense) in addition to your new group policy. A federal law called COBRA guarantees you the right to continue your group health insurance for at least eighteen months — but at your own cost. COBRA also gives you the right to continue your old policy, even after your new policy begins, if the new policy contains a pre-existing condition clause. You submit HIV-related claims on your "old" group policy until the pre-existing condition clause on the new policy no longer applies.

Use your "system-sense"; compare the system's objectives with your own. The insurance company's primary objective is *not* to pay your claims. It is *not* to protect your health or help you protect your health. These are *your* objectives. Their objective is to maintain profits by excluding "bad risks" from their customer base and rejecting as many claims as possible thereafter.

The pre-existing condition clause is a major weapon in the effort to reject claims. In using it, insurance companies look for direct and indirect evidence of pre-existing conditions. The T4 test, for example, is a red flag, because it's given only when something is seriously wrong. The insurance company doesn't care about the results. If they know you were tested, they can claim that you must have known or suspected you had HIV.

How would an insurance company know you took a T4 test? If you signed a release authorizing access to your medical records, you'll get caught. When applying for individual insurance policies, you must sign such a release. Information you've put on any insurance application may also have been forwarded to the Medical Information Bureau and then to your current insurance company.

The Medical Information Bureau (MIB) is a private, non-profit "trade association" of about eight hundred life and health insurance companies that maintains a centralized database of information collected from insurance applicants. (HMOs and Blue Cross Blue Shield are not members of the MIB.) Member companies submit a brief, coded summary to the MIB with the results of the underwriting evaluation of every insurance applicant. According to the MIB's rules, only information collected during an application for an insurance policy is reported to the MIB and this information is available only to member insurance companies, with written authorization from the consumer. Non-member companies and credit or consumer reporting agencies are not supposed to have access to MIB records. Medical conditions are reported to the MIB using over 200 codes. There are four medical codes that relate to HIV:

- "abnormal blood test for which there is no specific code" (the code used to report positive HIV test results);
- "abnormal T-cell study";
- "unexplained history of thrush, other opportunistic infections, weight loss, generalized chronic swelling of lymph nodes, persistent fever or diarrhea"; and
- "diagnosis of AIDS."

Information on claims made on life, health, or disability insurance is not supposed to be reported to the MIB. However, the MIB is private and self-policing — it enforces its own regulations. How would a consumer know if a violation occurred? A number of consumers claim they already have.

In 1981, a California man thought the MIB had obtained and released damaging claims information to a local insurance company. He went to court to obtain access to his MIB file — and failed. The MIB successfully argued that it does no business in California and cannot be sued in California courts, even though it maintains files on millions of Californians and releases that information to companies writing insurance policies in California (*Szabo v. MIB 1981*).

In Massachusetts, the MIB has been named in a number of complaints to the Massachusetts Commission Against Discrimination (MCAD). According to the executive director of the MCAD's AIDS Discrimination Hotline, many complaints were filed *before* HIV, particularly by cancer patients alleging they had been denied insurance coverage because the MIB had obtained and disseminated treatment information. More recently, the Boston chapter of ACT-UP has met with MIB officials to discuss complaints of HIV-infected people.

The Medical Information Bureau database also contains information about your lifestyle — again, to flag the bad risks.

When you applied for life insurance, for example, you may have found that your neighbors were quizzed about your life-style. Do you come home at night? What are your hobbies? Do you bring a lot of "overnight visitors" home and so forth. (They may even have a code for promiscuous and another code for homo ... and a very special code for both.)

Keeping HIV off the record is not enough. For example, a bout of shingles doesn't mean you have HIV. But if the insurance company finds out about the shingles you had last year, they can argue that, as a reasonable person who is a gay man, you should have suspected HIV and probably did get an HIV test. They don't have to prove you knew your HIV status. They can say, "We *assume* you did!" Worse, they can say, "You *should* have gotten tested!" Using either of these rationales, the insurance company could refuse to pay your HIV-related medical bills during the pre-existing condition period.

If you have an individual policy, your insurer can also refuse to pay your claims or can even cancel your policy if they can prove you did not complete an application correctly.

Imagine having to hire a lawyer when you're sick and need the coverage. Remember, the insurance company already has hired guns in its legal department.

Moreover, the insurance companies are getting ever more sophisticated in claiming what a reasonable person would think indicates HIV. Thrush, herpes, and shingles are all potential red flags. Even skin conditions, which commonly afflict people with HIV, can be cause for concern. *Try to keep HIV-related treatments off the record if you are insurance shopping or job hunting.*

Doctors are generally cooperative in this regard, but you must take the initiative. Doctors want to treat you. Since they understand that the insurance company's intent is to avoid paying for your treatment, they can get quite creative in terms of what they write in your record. (If your doctor doesn't want to help you, you have the wrong doctor.)

Surprisingly, there are certain times when you may want your HIV status to be recorded. For example, after you've been hired and *are safely past the probationary period when you can be dismissed without cause,* it can be advantageous to tell your employer's personnel department that you are HIV-positive. Having proof that your HIV status was known can help protect you, should you later contest a dismissal, layoff, or reassignment. The company must show it has not discriminated against you.

In sum, get group health and disability insurance policies. Understand the pre-existing condition clause in your policy. And know who is aware of the tests and treatments you take.

SINS OF OMISSION AND SINS OF COMMISSION: TALKING TO THE SYSTEM

We have been discussing choices you can make about withholding information. That's what Catholics call a Sin of Omission. There are also times when you need to consider Sins of Commission. In other words, *know when to lie.*

STOP RIGHT THERE, some of you may be saying. How can you *say* that? *Do you really mean lie?*

May I ask you how you've dealt with the following situations? Have you ever said any of the following:
- "You've lost weight!"
- "Oh, what a lovely gift!"
- "I'm sorry, I have a headache tonight."

Have you ever omitted information — or exaggerated...
- on a college financial aid application?
- on a tax return?
- on your resume?

HIV is a lot more important than these situations — but it doesn't work much differently. Consider the HIV-testing issue. In some areas, there is little or no anonymous testing. Only "confidential" testing is available. The lab or health center asks your name — and promises to keep the results confidential. If you were dependent on this system, would you use your real name? Or would you consider using a different name, say, "Dan Quayle"?

You might say that giving a false name to a lab is a fib, not a lie. It's small. Not very risky to you or harmful to anyone else. Lies may seem to be another, larger matter altogether. You are not supposed to lie.

The choices you make around HIV testing are choices about information: what information to share with the system, what information to withhold, and, maybe, when to lie. In the same way, the systems themselves make choices about information every day. Powerful people, organizations, and institutions bid for your attention, money, or support; in exchange they promise various benefits. Sometimes they exaggerate. Sometimes they omit key information. Sometimes (gasp) they tell outright falsehoods.

To refresh your memory and give you a chance to digest this point, consider the following well-known messages. How would you rate their truthfulness?

1	2	3	4	5
Pure truth	*Exaggeration*	*Fib*	*Lie*	*Satan said this*

- Pork, the other white meat!
- Ford has a better idea!
- It has not been proven that cigarette smoking is hazardous to your health. (Tobacco Industry Council, 1940–1980)
- I am not a crook. (Richard Nixon)
- Guns don't kill people, people do. (NRA)
- I don't recall... (Ronald Reagan)
- You're in good hands with Allstate.
- I never harassed her. (Clarence Thomas)
- I am not a racist. (David Duke)
- Read my lips. No new taxes. (George Bush)
- It's a great price! (Any realtor or car salesman)

You interact with systems all the time. Many of them are neither just nor truthful. If you're wealthy or well connected, this has never been a problem. You have ways of making the system work for you. If you have HIV and are *not* wealthy or well connected, you have some homework to do from now on.

System Law #2:
> *Know when the system is lying to you.*
> *Know when you have to lie to the system.*

FINANCIAL PROPHYLAXIS: GETTING DISABILITY INCOME INSURANCE

Prophylaxis is the medical term for preventive treatment. Financial prophylaxis is my term for the other great issue facing people with HIV: avoiding poverty. Health insurance does not suffice. One three-month illness could cost you your job and your savings. After successful treatment, you'd have your health back. But you would be poor and unemployable. Think what that kind of stress would do to your health.

You need disability income insurance to keep HIV from driving you into poverty. Besides, wouldn't you like the option of cutting back to part-time or not working at all some day? That's what disability insurance gives you. Once officially disabled, you not only collect on your group disability policy, you also collect Social Security Disability Income (SSDI) from the federal government. SSDI is one of the programs your FICA payroll taxes support.

Between your disability payment and SSDI, which kicks in six months later and is essentially not taxed, you could collect close to 80 percent of your current net pay. Your income on disability will not be great, but it may be adequate.

Let's examine how much *you* would collect on disability. The major variables are your salary and the payout level of your disability policy. Minor variables are state and local tax rates. Most disability policies will deduct your SSDI payments dollar for dollar, so that you collect exactly 60 percent of your pre-disability gross income, as specified by the policy.

The following worksheet illustrates how much someone making $30,000 would take home on a standard disability policy. Use the blank part of the worksheet to figure out how much *you* would collect on disability.

The financial advantages of disability insurance are obvious: When you can't work, your income will be protected. Less obvious are the benefits to your health. Many people find that once they stop working, their health improves. The stress of bad bosses or too much work is gone. Furthermore, getting disability insurance — or a job that offers it — will reduce your stress level right away. Worrying about your future is bad for your health *today*.

There are some details to attend to. As with health insurance, DI policies usually contain a pre-existing condition clause — generally one or two years. If you become disabled and stop working within that period, you won't receive any payments until the period is up. Unless you have a financial safety net, your job is to stay on the payroll and keep working until the pre-existing condition period is over.

SAMPLE WORKSHEET

	Before Disability	After Disability
Gross Income		
Salary	$30,000	0
Disability payment	0	10,000
SSDI (essentially not taxable)	0	8,000
Subtotal	30,000	18,000
Less		
Federal tax*	5,200	1,200
State/local tax	1,200	400
FICA (7%)	2,100	0
Subtotal	8,500	1,600
NET	**21,500**	**16,400**

*From federal tax tables; taxable gross income, less standard deduction

YOUR WORKSHEET

	Before Disability	After Disability
Gross Income		
Salary		
Disability payment		
SSDI (essentially not taxable)	_____	_____
Subtotal		
Less		
Federal tax		
State/local tax		
FICA (7%)		
Other	_____	_____
Subtotal		
NET		

Then there is the length of coverage — how long will the policy pay? Individual disability may pay out for two, three, or five years, or until age sixty-five. Group policies, on the other hand, generally pay out till you are sixty-five.

Finally, how long you collect also depends on a clause in your policy defining disability. [This is the fine print.] It's called the degree of disability clause. Pay attention to it.

On a group policy, the definition of *disabled* typically changes over time. In the first year you collect, disabled means not able to do your current job. In years two and three, by contrast, disabled may mean you're unable to perform a comparable job, appropriate to your skills and educational background. In later years, the definition becomes narrower still: It may mean you're unable to perform *any* job.

Over time, the insurance company will periodically review your case to see that you still qualify. It's your doctor who fills out the paperwork for these reviews. You must alert your doctor to the degree of disability provision and let him know what you need on that form. It's easy to show that you can't perform your current job. But four years later, maybe the insurance company will say you could be delivering newspapers or working at Burger King. Do you want to be working at Burger King?

You must alert your doctor *before* key events like a disability review. Especially as the criteria become more stringent, you must take care to note intangible concerns like fatigue, which contribute to disabling conditions and cannot easily be contested by the insurance company. The stress of worrying about losing your disability payments is real and harmful to your health. If you have established a good rapport with your doctor, he'll understand this. If he does not understand this, you don't have the right doctor *or* you haven't built a good relationship.

You won't be surprised to learn that my mother prepared me for this. A former World War II WAVE, Barbara was on veteran's disability for forty years. Prior to an annual disability review, I remember her putting on an old sweater and shuffling to the mirror, where she rumpled her clothes and smudged her lipstick a bit. When she thought I wasn't looking, she took a cigarette and burned a few well-placed holes. Then she was off to see her doctor. Barbara may have been crazy, but she wasn't stupid. Even after decades on disability, she took no chances with the review process.

I stopped working in February 1987, about a year after my diagnosis. To keep my lesions under control, I'd been juggling radiation and various chemotherapies, taking care to stop the treatment before damage was done. The treatments were effective for a few months — and then the lesions would start up again.

A month earlier I had started a new chemotherapy, interferon, and I wasn't feeling well. I decided to just work less and less frequently — and finally not at all — and see what happened. After six weeks, someone in Personnel caught on and activated the short-term disability policy. Three months later, when I had not returned to work, my long-term disability policy was activated. I was officially disabled. My disability company sent me a detailed letter showing how much I would receive every year — until the year 2015, when I would turn sixty-five and convert to Social Security. (Now *here's* a system, I thought.)

Disability was a mixed bag at first. I knew it was good for my health, since my job at Yankee had become quite dull and I didn't need the stress of juggling work and interferon treatments. But I was concerned that not working meant I was giving up. I wanted to keep working part-time — but on my own schedule and on projects I truly enjoyed. My disability policy allowed me to return to part-time work at Yankee without losing my benefits, once I had been out on disability a few months. But I couldn't imagine a suitable part-time position there. If I left Yankee for another employer, I would lose all my benefits.

The solution? I decided to volunteer at my AIDS service organization. In March, I called Taffy, my Advocate, who said he would pass my request along. Perhaps he did — or perhaps it went to Never-Never Land. For the next six months, I focused on stabilizing my health.

BUILD RAPPORT WITH PEOPLE IN THE SYSTEM

You need allies in the HIV system — insiders who are also your partners. Your doctor should be one of those people.

If you had met your doctor just this afternoon and wanted to get on disability, he would run batteries of tests before writing your disability letter. If you've known him a while and have a good relationship, however, he'll want to help you and will ask, "What needs to go in the letter?" That's the kind of rapport you want with your doctor.

Building rapport with insiders is up to you. The doctors won't think they have the time for it. Nor have they been trained for it. Building rapport also takes planning and commitment on your part.

As a college student, I generally paid an office visit to my professors near the end of the semester. I would make up a question and ask them to clarify the subject for me. "Thank you, thank you," I murmured gratefully, knowing that when grading time came, if my grade were on the cusp between a C+ and a B-, the professor would be likely to give me the benefit of the doubt.

In daily life, we build rapport with insiders all the time. Think about restaurants. Who is the insider you want as an ally? The waiter, of course.

Some people don't see the waiter as an ally. On a busy night, when the harried waiter approaches, they grumble, "Go get me some water. I've been sitting here for ten minutes!" Other people might say, "Gee, you're terribly busy. You'd think your boss would have more people on tonight! We're not in a hurry. When you get a chance, could you get me some water?"

Guess who gets the water faster?

Why would you want an ally at a restaurant? Not just to get your water quickly. You want to know what's the best thing on the menu today. If you curse the waiter, he might not give you the best advice. You might find yourself ordering the Chicken Salmonella Special!

So you're nice to people.

With medical staff, start out on the right foot by showing interest in them as people. Ask where they live, whether they're new to the area, family details, and so forth. The rapport must go both ways. Let the staff know you're an intelligent human being — more than a collection of symptoms connected to labels on test tubes! How do you do that? By talking about your medical care and other things you're interested in.

If you build an adult relationship — a partnership —

with your doctor, the payoff is significant. You get better communication and cooperation — and that means better care. Doctors are people. They can be influenced. Your doctor should *want* to write you a disability letter. Or get you that experimental drug. Or untangle a snafu with another department.

SOCIAL SERVICE SYSTEMS: KNOW WHAT TO EXPECT

People with HIV deal with many systems: medical facilities, insurance companies, and AIDS service organizations. After organizing my medical care and attending to disability, the next system I had to tackle was Boston's AIDS service organization, the AIDS Action Committee of Massachusetts.

People with HIV often approach ASOs with greater hopes and aspirations than other HIV bureaucracies. After all, ASOs have community roots, including staff and volunteers living with HIV. They are not entrenched, like government agencies or insurance companies. And they specialize in HIV. However, AIDS organizations *are* systems, like hospitals and insurance companies. They have moving parts and they make errors. Unlike hospitals and other agencies, AIDS organizations haven't had a century or more to delineate roles and procedures.

Consider, for a moment, where these organizations come from. They were started from scratch by volunteers and they were constructed rapidly. The oldest organization, New York's Gay Men's Health Crisis, was just ten years old in 1992. ASOs have grown and changed on a scale that dwarfs anything in the private sector: exploding caseloads, rapid invention and proliferation of programs, and high turnover of staff and volunteers due to burnout and illness. All the while, they faced a continuously changing kaleidoscope of treatments, funding, and government policies.

When I first asked for services in 1986 and 1987, I had a hard time. Things fell between the cracks in odd ways.

My contact at AIDS Action was Taffy, a client advocate. Early on, I asked him for literature on the pros and cons of chemotherapy versus radiation. Instead of medical information, Taffy sent me brochures about macrobiotic diets and connected me to a support group.

Hmm, I thought. *Is this how it's supposed to work?*

The following spring, as I was winding up my interferon therapy, I began investigating AZT. Wondering if it might work better in conjunction with chemotherapy, I asked Taffy, "Can you tell me where to get information on AZT and chemotherapy?"

"I don't have that information, Bob," he replied.

"That's okay. I wouldn't expect anyone to have it at their fingertips."

I paused, waiting for him to suggest something. There was a long silence at the other end of the line. I continued.

"What can you do to get that information?"

"Why would I know how to get that kind of information?"

"Because then you could tell *me* how to get it. And I could find out what to do about my health!" Wasn't this how the system was supposed to work?

After another silence, Taffy apologized and changed the subject. He had complementary tickets to the Whitney Houston concert. Would I like to go? Incredulous, I said no. Taffy clearly did not think of his job the way I did.

Something is wrong here, I thought to myself. *When I ask for medical information, I get advice about granola and tickets to rock concerts.* I tried contacting Taffy's boss, without success, wondering if I had the right expectations. At the same time, I was careful to keep things positive with Taffy. He was often quite droll and we enjoyed a bit of banter.

Today, AIDS organizations hire client advocates with more skills and experience than Taffy and give them some medical training, but they often lag behind the complexities of the epidemic. If you find a service provider's behavior puzzling, try talking with him about his expectations:

- What kind of services can I expect from your agency?
- What is your assessment of my needs at this point?
- How do my needs compare with other clients you serve?
- Which services can you help me with?
- Who else can I see to get services?
- How can I help you serve me better?
- What if I have a problem?

(Had I done this, I might have learned that Taffy had a caseload of sixty and was, on his own and with no support, spearheading outreach in the Haitian community, even though he spoke no Creole.)

I also encountered a lack of follow-through. The left hand didn't know what the right was doing. For example, I requested an emotional support volunteer, called a buddy. Taffy passed the request along to someone. A few months later, I asked when I would receive my buddy. Taffy didn't know.

"Is my name on a list?"

He didn't know that either.

I started to realize that AIDS organizations were systems, too — and that I did not know how they worked. I wondered if Taffy himself knew. As I pondered these system errors, I became intrigued. In the fall of 1987, I read that AIDS Action was growing rapidly, with nearly forty staff and a thousand volunteers in dozens of different programs. I realized I could offer a lot as a volunteer. Designing information systems was my specialty, after all. I know how to fix these problems, I thought to myself.

By Thanksgiving of 1987, I felt well enough to volunteer. I asked Taffy again to put me in touch with the volunteer program. Over a year had elapsed since my first request.

This time I found a way into the system. The volunteer experience itself was surprising and unconventional. It expanded my horizons and improved my ability to manage my health. I got inside the system and found not only the information I needed, but sustenance as well. In particular, I made three friends whom I need to talk about here.

In February 1988, I got a call from the volunteer director, Michael Connolly. I told him I had AIDS, was on long-term disability, was a systems analyst, and wanted to volunteer. He invited me to a March meeting of information systems volunteers. I arrived at AIDS Action a few weeks later, carrying my resume. I was both skeptical and anxious as I walked down a maze of narrow halls to a small office crammed with four desks. *Their turf,* I thought.

I was greeted by a tall man with sandy brown hair, a mustache, a nice tie — and no shoes. I shook his hand and said, "Hi. I'm Bob Rimer. I brought you my resume."

"Thanks," said Michael, tossing my resume onto a stack of papers, "I'll show you to the meeting." I thought he was utterly distracted.

The room was crowded with people and computers. On the walls were colorful sheets of newsprint outlining programs and objectives. That seemed interesting. A volunteer spoke about using computers to improve various services and the group debated what kind of questionnaire to send to staff. This bored me. Half of these people are cruising each other, I thought. They're not thinking this through.

After a while, I spoke up. "Nobody answers question-naires," I offered. "You need to talk to staff in person. It's more practical and it will help you sell yourselves and your pro-gram." Some people agreed; some did not. The conversation about the questionnaire continued.

Beneath the newsprint sat a short, spectacled man wearing a colorful bow tie. As the meeting adjourned, he raised his eye-brows and pointed a stubby arm at me. "Who ... are ... you?" It was Larry Killian, director of the Finance and Information Sys-tems Department. We chatted briefly. "Look," I explained, "com-puterization is not about wires and computers. It's about how people work with each other and talk with each other."

"Absolutely!" he concurred, and he invited me out for a drink — to interview me. He asked about my background and skills and told me about his own. He'd run a bookstore in Vermont and directed marketing for publishing companies in Boston before coming to AIDS Action in 1985. Since then, he had launched a blizzard of finance and fundraising programs. He was engaging, provocative, and buoyantly cynical.

He was also extremely creative. Recently he'd formatted the annual budget as a trip down the Grand Canyon. "No one ever reads budgets," he explained, "especially not human services types. My goal is just to get them to look at the damn thing."

I thought of Taffy trying to read a budget — or ride a raft down the Colorado. Maybe I couldn't work so well with Taffy, but I knew I could work with Larry Killian. (Partner #1: Found and Hired.) I offered to turn the computer volunteers into a professional Management Information Systems (MIS) depart-ment composed of both staff and volunteers. I would work three days a week.

Larry was concerned. "That's a big responsibility. Will your health permit it?"

This question irked me. Was I going to be discounted again? "I'll bet the typical employee is only here a year or two,"

I countered. "I'll be around that long. If I get sick, I'll work from home."

"Fine. Then make next Monday your first day."

At last. A doorway was opening into the system. On Monday, I learned more.

AIDS Action was building partnerships with other agencies. It was lobbying, training, and sometimes funding them to deliver HIV-related services that AIDS Action itself could not provide. Internally, all staff were to become volunteer managers. I saw that a good computer network would allow staff and volunteers to get more work done more accurately — without hiring as many new staff.

Later, at home, I drafted a proposal for a Management Information Systems (MIS) department with two full-time staff and a dozen volunteers. When I came in bearing my proposal on Wednesday, Larry was setting up computer equipment.

"Something's wrong with this," he sighed. "Do you know anything about printers?"

"I don't know anything about plugs and wires," I replied. "I'm not a hardware person; I'm a consultant." I handed him my proposal.

"I see ... I don't suppose you'll be wanting a computer on your desk?"

"No, I don't use them."

"Great," he chortled. "I have an Information Systems volunteer who won't touch computers! That may not work around here, Bob."

A couple of hours later, he returned my proposal, heavily annotated. I'd overlooked a number of issues. "I like it," he said, "but it needs work. We're hiring our first full-time computer person in August. People will ask why we should hire a second one, rather than an additional advocate."

I liked the prompt feedback. This guy takes me seriously! "I'll show them the logic," I replied. "Organizing the computer group properly will actually allow advocates to do more for clients — as much as hiring three new staff."

Larry looked over his glasses. "Sounds awfully easy."

"I'll get buy-in during my needs assessment interviews. Wait and see." I ticked off key decision makers whom I planned to see. Larry added several names to my list. I was under way.

Larry also asked me to manage telephone operations for a few months. The administrative director, Connie, was pregnant and would be leaving the agency. Telecommunications and Office Management would become part of Larry's Finance Department. At the same time, AIDS Action was preparing to move to new, larger quarters at the end of the summer. A new phone system was needed and, possibly, a new voicemail system.

I met Connie. She was preparing to buy an expensive phone system and didn't even have an up-to-date staff and volunteer telephone directory.

Afterwards, I asked Larry, "Does Connie have trouble distinguishing the more important from the less important?" He grinned and suggested I work directly with Connie's assistant, Michelle, on the phone directory. Michelle worked on the directory in fits and starts — names, titles, extensions, voicemail codes. I caught errors on her first attempt. The next two attempts were worse. The fourth one looked okay. I gave it to Larry.

"She left out an entire department," he pointed out.

I handed it back to her. "Michelle, this list still has errors."

She was incensed. Her vacation was due to begin in two days. "Larry Killian asked me to do that," she harrumphed. "Well, I did it and I'm done!"

Then she turned her back to me and said derisively, "You're just an uppity volunteer."

I began to steam. Putting my hands on my hips, I said loudly, "I am appalled that you are drawing a paycheck!" People peeked around various partitions.

In frustration, I retreated to Larry's office, sputtering, "How can people be so stupid!"

His eyes twinkled. "I inherited her three weeks ago. And her title is office manager. There is no secretary in my department."

"If she can't manage a phone list, she obviously can't manage an office! Why don't you fire her?"

"Bob, you'll have to learn how things work here. That's not the process." He had me photocopy the erroneous work and attach an explanation. Then it went into a file he'd already prepared. I wondered what other piles of doody I would soon be stepping in.

Michelle may or may not have been a bad hire. That's not

important. What is important are the dynamics of the system. I saw staff in transition from jobs they hadn't mastered to jobs that hadn't been defined. I also realized the staff had mixed feelings about volunteers — and about people with HIV. Meanwhile, demands on the agency were increasing and new programs were ramping up. There were a lot of balls in the air.

As summer of 1988 began, I interviewed a dozen managers and board members, explaining to them how computers could help them do their jobs. For the most part, they impressed me. I began to realize that AIDS Action was a very smart beast — but one with six heads, moving in several directions at once. It was far more complicated than Yankee Atomic. And I had to admit, the staff worked far harder and were very talented. They were fixing and improving things faster than any private company — but the epidemic kept outpacing them.

Over the course of the summer, I got more involved. I presented my assessment to the management team. They bought the goals and concepts, but said no to the second computer person, at least until the following year. I was to use volunteers and business-school interns. I was also asked to help hire the MIS manager and to begin attending a volunteer coordinating committee, which elected the board of directors.

Larry Killian, in particular, I came to worship. We operated in true partnership. He managed me, but was willing to be managed *by* me as well. He was the least egocentric boss I'd ever had — and the smartest. He struck me as Einstein on mescaline.

I liked my new job!

In September, Larry was tested for HIV. For months he'd been plagued by a series of rashes and bumps and now fevers. The results were positive. I was devastated. A week later, a nasty flu grounded him and set the stage for my partnerships with Larry's closest friends on staff, David Aronstein and Michael Connolly.

With Michael, Larry was to present several management workshops at a national conference for AIDS staff and volunteers. Two days before the conference, Larry asked me to take his place. I said yes, but was uneasy, since I was accustomed to presenting project plans, not management theory.

"Don't worry — we can do this," said Michael. He quickly

reviewed the outlines for two workshops and promised to help me draft the third after we got to New Orleans. Once there, he took me for a trolley ride through the Garden District, to Tulane University, where we got stoned and chatted about family heroes and misfits. Michael had worked for years with retarded people before getting an MBA. After some marketing and teaching, he'd volunteered for Larry in 1986 and came on staff as the director of volunteers the next year.

"Why did it take me a year to get a call about volunteering?" I asked him, remembering how he tossed aside my resume.

"That's a success, Bob! When you gave your name to Taffy in 1986, it probably went into a volunteer's shoe box, if he gave it to anyone at all. No one even knew how many volunteers there were. Now we respond to everyone who sends in an application, but it takes months."

I told him about my early efforts to work the AIDS Action system. I found that Larry had been reporting to Michael about me daily. They had been giggling for months about my encounters with the system.

"I like absurdity and surprises," Michael mused.

"And I'm attracted to dysfunction!" I confessed. "It arouses me."

"Welcome aboard!" he said drily. I'd found my second ally. "Introducing systems here has been very tricky," he continued. "People come here to cause change. Then, when change starts to happen, they get upset and dig in their heels! You've got your work cut out for you. If you want to change the client services system, get to know David Aronstein. He moved mountains to build it." Then we returned to the hotel. The workshops went well.

Later, at a crowded cocktail party, I sidled up to David. As we surveyed the crowd picking at tired canapés, I suggested, "Maybe we should go to a restaurant."

"I'd like a *nice* meal," said David cautiously.

"I don't care what it costs!" I blurted. David's face brightened and we were off. Over an elegant dinner, we struck up a rapport.

"Why," I asked, "do client services staff have trouble with requests for medical information?"

"Many clients face crises," he pointed out. "Evictions,

firings, drug problems. When you're focusing on those things, it's hard to keep up with medical stuff."

"How come Taffy didn't know if the buddy program kept a list of clients waiting for service?"

He shrugged. "Taffy was one of our earlier hires."

"Is he the only one with this problem?"

"Not really. Look, I built this department fast. It outgrew me — and some of the advocates, too."

"Why don't you fire the incompetent ones?"

"I can't fire them all, Bob!" he parried.

I was tickled. David had a sense of humor and was not defensive. I had found my third ally. The three of them — Larry, Michael, and David — I thought of as the Three Musketeers.

When we returned to Boston, Larry was recovering from the flu. David became director of a new Policy and Planning group. Michael was working with volunteers — particularly people with HIV — to organize a medical library and weekly PWA dinners, which I began attending. I realized I could get the medical information I needed without going through client advocates.

Michael joked to me, "I get the squeaky wheel clients to come in and run the agency. Besides the buddy program, volunteering is one opportunity we offer clients that I know works!"

Meanwhile, a new client services director was hired, a burly man whom I'll refer to as Earl. With a team of new volunteers, I began organizing a two-year project to give client advocates access to computerized information about their caseload, and about services available throughout Massachusetts.

As 1988 ended, my frame of reference had changed dramatically. I'd found a way past the moving parts, into my AIDS organization, where I now had a title, a desk, and a boss. I had challenging projects and was meeting very knowledge-able people with HIV. I was getting the information I needed to continue towards my goals and I was making a difference.

I also had the Three Musketeers. I did not know they would soon be far more than allies in a system. They would become dear friends.

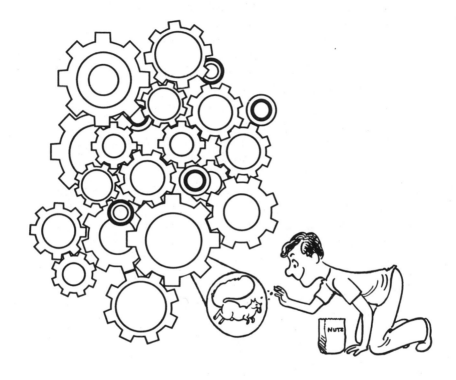

MORAL: **Understand the HIV bureaucracy by watching all the moving parts.**
What you don't know WILL eventually hurt you.

WORKING THE SYSTEM
Use this worksheet to see how these concepts might apply to you.

1. What do I have in place now?

_____an income I can count on

_____a doctor

_____group health insurance

_____group disability income insurance

_____T4 cell count

_____someone I can talk to

_____someone who already knows about HIV systems

2. What are my objectives as of today?

3. What do I need to work on first?

4. What are my own skills and resources?

3

Monitoring
Your Health

Monitoring your health is like driving a car. You constantly check for two things: that the car is running well, and that you're on a safe course.

When the oil meter flashes low, most people check the oil and add more. Some people, however, don't do the small, simple things. They don't like checking the oil. They ignore warning lights. Pretty soon, BOOM, the engine seizes up! My brother Stevie has lost four cars this way.

To stay on course, drivers do a number of simple things, like looking in the rearview mirror, staying between the white lines, checking the speedometer, and letting up on the brake. Drivers constantly make small adjustments.

After HIV, you need to manage your body at least as thoughtfully as your car. You must attend to small changes before they turn into big problems.

Because doctors administer lots of tests to people with HIV, you may think they are monitoring your health. WRONG. *You* monitor your health and treat yourself on a daily basis — *not* your doctor. Your doctor spends as much time with you as your auto mechanic does with your car — and feels about as secure in her knowledge. The tests give her important clues about your health, but they are no substitute for firsthand knowledge.

You, on the other hand, have "operated" your body for decades. You know your body's unique *personality*. You've watched it perform under adverse conditions. You've conducted routine maintenance and made midcourse corrections. If your body were a valuable machine, you would have kept a written maintenance log.

Working with your doctor, you can harvest this experience and monitor your health. Just as before you had HIV, you want to spot little problems early and fix them before they get bigger.

Here are some of the questions you're probably thinking about:

- How can I stay healthy?
- How do I know when something is serious?
- How do I know what to do first?
- What do I ask my doctor?
- What if I don't agree with my doctor?
- How do I know when my doctor is doing more harm than good?

The trick is to remember your body's personality, avoid stressful events and procedures, and try simple solutions first.

NOT EVERYTHING IS HIV-RELATED

Not every illness you get after HIV is a major deal. *People with HIV catch common colds, too.*

If you had a weak point before HIV, it's still there. If you got earaches as a little kid, you will do so after HIV — and they won't be any more HIV-related than they ever were. Furthermore, just because you're getting sick doesn't mean you won't get better! Intellectually, you may know you'll get better. In the back of your mind, however, may be the fear that "this is it." This is not an earache — it's a brain tumor. It's going to get worse and worse. "Here I go!"

Even if you manage to keep your own paranoia to a minimum, your friends or lover may still succumb.

My weak point has always been upper respiratory. Eyes, ears, nose, throat. In the summer of 1988, a couple of months after I started volunteering at AIDS Action, I had an earache. It came on swiftly and painfully one afternoon. The next morning I was too dizzy to drive, so Mario had to take me to the hospital — for the first time since my diagnosis. He was more nervous than I was — and managed to "tap" a car in front of us. I haven't asked him to take me to the hospital since and he hasn't offered. It's better this way for both of us.

As I didn't have a primary care physician, I went to Oncology, where I usually saw Bubbles, and spoke to a nurse.

"I need ampicillin. I have an ear infection and it really hurts."

The nurse was alarmed. "We should take a look first, Bob. We don't really know what it is!" she said. "It could be any number of things. Perhaps KS!"

"Yes," I conceded, "it could be. But I've been getting earaches since I was a little boy. I have problems with my ears. Why don't you just give me ampicillin. I bet this will clear up. And if it doesn't, then I'll come talk to you."

She checked with Bubbles, who wrote me an ampicillin prescription. Bubbles knew by now that I didn't jump to conclusions.

"You should start to feel better within forty-eight hours," stressed the nurse. "If you don't, call me."

I took the ampicillin and of course the earache went away. The lesson I draw from this is: Not everything is HIV-related.

The nurse, on the other hand, was trained in oncology. She was looking for that 2 percent probability that my earache indicated some kind of cancer. It was her job to err on the side of caution, rather than overlook something that might be serious. From my perspective, however, poking around in my ear or cutting a slice off for a biopsy were not things to rush into!

When a person with HIV gets a bad headache, the doctor wants to diagnose it correctly. She has a list of thirty horrible things that could be the cause. But chances are, it's the same migraine or stress-related headache you used to get. Or a little ear infection. Similarly, if you have a sore throat, you may have a cold or your mouth may have been somewhere it shouldn't have been. *Just like before you knew you were HIV-positive.*

So what do you do? You gargle with hot salty water, take aspirin, and sleep off your cold. You don't start out by having them stick a tube into your lungs and take a little snip for a biopsy. The doctors, on the other hand, may want to cut you open to biopsy you, on the small chance that something more serious really is going on.

Before assuming that a health problem is HIV-related, consider simpler causes. Don't panic.

AVOIDING INVASIVE PROCEDURES

Doctors know that trauma is bad for the body. In hospitals, trauma means broken bones, gunshot wounds, cuts and gashes — *some of them administered by doctors themselves.* For example, knee operations used to require ten days of recovery in the hospital. A new procedure called arthroscopy has eliminated 98 percent of the trauma. Instead of slicing open the whole knee, a fiberoptic tube is inserted into a tiny hole and — snip snip — the cutting and splicing of tendons is quickly done in the doctor's office. Virtually no trauma. And no bed rest needed afterwards!

I believe trauma is particularly harmful to people with HIV.

Even changes in routine can be traumatic. For example, sleeping in a new bed at a guest house, or big changes in my diet, or staying up all night — all of which I tolerated quite well before HIV — cause minor health problems now. And invasive procedures are far worse. They can aggravate existing health problems or trigger new ones.

What do I mean by "invasive procedure"? I mean invading the body. Cutting you open or putting a tube where your body doesn't want a tube: bronchoscopies, colonoscopies, endoscopies, biopsies, and rectal exams (unless you like them).

Invasive procedures have a cost. Sometimes it is small; sometimes it is large. For people with HIV, the cost often outweighs the benefit. You must be the judge.

I learned this the hard way. My first lesson was in June 1986. I had been diagnosed with KS three months earlier and was experiencing bowel problems. Dr. Clean, my oncologist, wanted to check for internal lesions, so he sent me down to Internal Medicine for a colonoscopy. During a colonoscopy, a thin, five-foot-long fiberoptic tube is threaded into your colon. It's frightening and uncomfortable. Most people require Valium beforehand and bed rest after. I was given Valium.

The view was transmitted to a television screen above me. It revealed a few internal lesions. That was the benefit. The colonoscopy gave my doctors useful information. They decided my current course of chemotherapy was adequate — more aggressive measures were not needed.

The benefit came at a cost: The colonoscopy was painful and stressful. It was also a shock to my system. Shortly thereafter, I had a herpes flare-up, which might have been an additional cost of the colonoscopy, since I had never had herpes before.

I was experiencing two kinds of trauma — the invasive procedure and stressful events. As you can imagine, this was a pretty stressful period. I had been diagnosed with AIDS, was given nine months to live, had just moved into a new house with Mario, and was starting chemotherapy. Then I had the colonoscopy. Bingo, I had rectal herpes two weeks later.

It started one Saturday morning in early July. The pain was excruciating, perhaps the worst pain I had ever experienced. Monday morning, I left an urgent message for Dr. Clean. Tuesday afternoon, when he had not returned my call, I called again, hysterical. Clean was too busy to speak with me. Jane, the nurse, told me just to come in.

I managed to see Clean, who put on rubber gloves and told me he wanted to do a rectal exam.

I knew this would be too painful. I had to generate some options or at least be certain that this was an ordeal I absolutely had to face. Forget it. Even then I didn't want to face it. As far as I was concerned, "no pain" would be a very big gain. I was motivated to be very creative.

Questions flashed through my mind.

Why does he want to do this?

Where will this take us? What will we learn?

Do I really want to go there?

Are there other ways to get there?

"You can't!" I exclaimed. "It's too painful. I can't let you put your finger in there. No way!"

He took another look and said, "I'll do a culture for herpes."

"Does it look like herpes?" I asked.

"I can't really tell," he replied. "It could be."

"How long does the test take?"

"About a week."

"A week! I have to live with this pain for a week? Can't you give me something in the meantime?"

He shrugged. "I could give you codeine, I suppose."

"Why can't you just treat me for herpes?"

"I don't know yet if you have herpes."

I paused before continuing. "How often, when you have herpes, will the test show you have herpes?"

"About 50 percent of the time," he responded. "It's actually a rather difficult virus to culture."

"What would you do if the culture did not show any herpes?"

"I would probably go ahead and treat you with acyclovir, the herpes medicine."

"Does it have any side effects?"

"No, it's quite safe."

"So let me get this straight. If I test negative, you'll give me acyclovir. What are you going to do if I test positive?"

"Oh, I'd treat you with acyclovir," he told me.

BINGO! I thought. No need to let his fingers do the walking. Just a little "scrip" writing would do nicely, thank you.

"Well, why don't you go ahead and give me the acyclovir now?"

Clean thought for a few seconds and said reluctantly, "Yeah, that makes sense!" He wrote a prescription for acyclovir, which I promptly filled. Within forty-eight hours I felt better.

In fact, the test later came back negative, perhaps because, as Clean had said, herpes was difficult to culture. In any event, we can assume from my response to the acyclovir that I had either herpes or a similar virus that acyclovir gets rid of.

We had avoided the trauma of an invasive procedure and tried simpler things first. We kept stress to a minimum. After all, it was probably stress and trauma that caused the problem in the first place. No pain. Big gain.

TREAT THINGS EMPIRICALLY

My motto is:

Try simpler things first.

Sometimes that means trying medication before being sure of the diagnosis, as when Clean treated my herpes with acyclovir. Sometimes modifying your current medication is enough. Other times it has nothing to do with drugs. You must define and weigh the options. Here's one example.

The spring following my colonoscopy and herpes adventures, my bowel problems returned. I was really straining to move my bowels — once a week! You can imagine how cranky I was. Like Leona Helmsley stuck at a Howard Johnson's.

Dr. Clean told me, "There might be more KS in there. We should take a look."

I was in no mood for this. "What are you looking for?" I asked.

"More KS."

"What will you do if you find it?"

"There's really not much more we can do than what we're doing right now," he said regretfully.

"Well," I said, "we knew KS was there last summer. Do you think it's gone away?"

"No."

"Are you looking for more of it?"

"Well, it might be spreading."

"So what are you going to do?"

"Nothing different from what I'm doing now."

"Then what difference would it make?"

"I just think we should know," he said earnestly.

He just wasn't going to let go. Okay. No more Mr. Nice Guy.

I sighed. "You said you're not going to treat me any differently. What is this obsession you have with my asshole?!"

(I said I was cranky!)

I knew Dr. Clean wanted to be thorough. But I wasn't about to undergo a painful colonoscopy and risk another herpes flare-up unless there were significant potential benefits. Clean couldn't articulate any benefits to me.

I wanted a simpler solution — definitely not just the first one that "routine procedures" brought to the medical mind. In fact, it is a rule of creative problem-solving to always consider at least three alternatives before deciding on any one — particularly not the first one. In this case, I was willing to settle for almost any alternative.

I had started taking interferon and had stopped working at the start of 1987. I wasn't willing to go back to work, but I thought maybe I could alter my relationship with interferon.

I continued. "We know constipation can be a side effect of interferon. Why don't we cut back the dose and see what happens?"

We did and my bowels returned to normal. The problem had been the drugs I was taking.

At the end of June, Dr. Clean transferred to another hospital. Bubbles, his boss, told me, "Just make your appointments with me from now on." I would continue to see Bubbles for two years.

Earlier I described how Bubbles prescribed ampicillin for my earache. He was treating me *empirically*. When the ampicillin made the earache go away, we knew I'd had bacteria in my ears. Because the medication had no harmful side effects, Bubbles had me try it, without waiting for the results of a culture. This wasn't routine procedure, but it worked for me.

When the medicine *does* have negative side effects, you must weigh them against the negative side effects of an invasive procedure. Sometimes doctors omit this step. That's why you must be monitoring everything. Before you agree to an invasive procedure or a powerful medication, you must ask *Why?* then ask again: Is there another way?

Here's another example.

Late the following year, 1988, my new AIDS Action boss, Larry Killian, thought he might have pneumocystis pneumonia (PCP). Two months earlier he had learned he was HIV-positive. And now he was getting sick. He was exhausted, had fevers, gasped from shortness of breath, and could not walk up a flight of stairs without resting.

At that time, the treatments for PCP were Bactrim and pentamidine, very strong medications with unpleasant side effects. Larry's doctor did not want to administer either unless he absolutely had to — unless he was sure Larry had PCP. To get a definitive diagnosis the doctor administered an invasive procedure called a bronchoscopy. A "bronch" is painful: A tube goes up your nose, then down the back of your throat into your lungs, where it takes a little snip. If you have PCP, the bronch will show it about 60 percent of the time. But not always. In 1988, the procedure was to try a second or third time.

I urged Larry to avoid the bronch. He and his doctor decided otherwise.

The first bronchoscopy revealed nothing abnormal, so Larry underwent a second one, even as he was getting sicker. He promptly had a major herpes flare-up on his lips and in his mouth and throat. ("I know, I know. You told me so.") Eventually his doctor treated him with Bactrim and Larry recovered — so the doctor concluded Larry had indeed had PCP.

Since that time, many doctors have decided that the side

effects of the bronchoscopy are worse than those of Bactrim. Now they don't wait for a definitive diagnosis to begin treatment. When they see clear PCP symptoms, they treat you *empirically*. In other words, they administer PCP medicine and wait. If your condition improves rapidly, they know you must have had PCP.

As you can see, it's not always easy to treat conditions empirically — nor is it necessarily the doctor's first preference. It's up to you to work with your doctor on this point. Sometimes the problem is not the doctor's attitude. Here's another example.

In the summer of 1990, I experienced headaches, short-term memory problems, and confusion.

"What could this be?" I wondered. I made an appointment with Millie, who's been my primary care physician since 1989, when my needs got more intense and Bubbles got too busy.

Dementia and depression were the obvious possibilities. Dementia is difficult to diagnose early, but a brain scan using MRI will sometimes reveal dementia when it's under way. Millie ordered an MRI in October for that reason. My brain looked perfectly normal.

At the same time, I had my therapist looking for depression. He didn't think it was depression, although my symptoms were suggestive. My therapist and Millie talked to each other and couldn't figure out the problem. We were checking out both possibilities and coming up dry.

Meanwhile, Millie had ordered a syphilis screening as part of a routine battery of blood tests. Three days before Christmas she telephoned me at home.

"You tested positive for syphilis. You're probably having a recurrence of syphilis from fifteen years ago." She was holding my public health records in front of her. "This condition is called neurological syphilis," she continued.

"How high was the titre?" I asked. (The *titre* is the level of antigen or infection measured in your system. Remember this word. You will hear it a lot.) I knew the count goes up steeply over the first two weeks of an active syphilis infection.

She gave me a reasonably low number.

"Why don't we take the test again in a few days?" I said. "The number should be going up very quickly if I have syphilis."

"We can't wait!" she said. "I want you in the hospital today. We need to do a spinal tap. I want to take care of this immediately."

Actually, she was about to leave for the Bahamas, so she was anxious to get this under control fast. On the other hand, I was pretty leery of spinal taps. Although I'd never had one, I knew several people who recalled spinal taps as *excruciating*. I told Millie so.

"They're not as bad as all that, Bob," she reassured me. "We have a really good doctor here."

"How do we know we'll get that doctor!" I asked. "Everyone I know who's had a spinal tap got *severe* headaches. For days! They couldn't even get out of bed! Besides," I added, "I heard that people with HIV have false positives on syphilis tests. Maybe my test results are wrong. Do you think that's a possibility here?"

"You're just being difficult!"

"Maybe. But I don't want that spinal tap if I can avoid it. Tell you what. I want to do a little research quickly. I'll call you back in an hour."

I jumped in my car and drove over to AIDS Action, where I called up on the computer all articles mentioning both HIV and syphilis. There were several.

I learned that false positives are indeed a problem for people with HIV. But here is what I also learned.

In a spinal tap, the doctor removes some of your CSF — cerebrospinal fluid — for analysis. In my case, they would look for syphilis germs. If the patient is HIV-infected and has neurological syphilis, half the time they do find syphilis, half the time they don't. In other words, the spinal fluid can falsely test *negative*. If they find active syphilis they treat you with fourteen days on intravenous penicillin.

And if they don't find the syphilis, they still treat you for syphilis.

I got back on the phone to Millie and read this portion of the article aloud.

"They're saying the spinal tap has a high rate of false negatives. Why not just treat me for syphilis?" I asked.

"That's not the procedure," she admonished. "Besides, we might find other things while doing the tap. This is serious stuff, Bob!"

"What could you find?"

"I don't know," she sputtered, "but Infectious Disease says we need to do a spinal tap."

We dickered for a while. I insisted on time to make more phone calls and continue reading the articles. Then I read about false positives. People with HIV sometimes show active syphilis on blood tests when they don't have it. I discussed this news with a medical case manager at a private company serving people with HIV. She confirmed it. I thought back to Julio and my numerous encounters with the elves in the blood lab. There was more than one reason why the blood test could be erroneous. I called Millie again.

"I have an article here that says people with HIV show false positives. Why don't we try the syphilis test again? You know the lab as well as I do."

Millie was irate.

I insisted. "It will only take twenty-four hours."

So I went in and we did the test again. The next day the results came back non-reactive. Negative. I did not have neurological syphilis. Millie was flabbergasted.

"I called Public Health," she told me, "and they said they've never encountered this situation before."

"That disturbs me even more, Millie!" I replied. "The articles I read said it's rather common!"

I was not faulting her medical logic. She could well have been right. My concern was that the spinal tap was so invasive that it might trigger other health problems. I wanted to do the simple things first, before undertaking invasive procedures. In this case, that meant repeating the blood test.

"So," said Millie, "what do you think is wrong? My hypothesis is HIV dementia. What is yours? We've ruled out syphilis and depression. What's left! This is serious. We need to do something!"

By coincidence, the media were at this very time reporting stories about the sleeping medication Halcion, which I had been taking daily for five years. Some people on high doses were getting psychotic and shooting their spouses. Others had severe confusion and memory loss.

I did not appear psychotic. Obstreperous, maybe, but not psychotic. (No one knew how often I thought of shooting Mario.) My confusion and memory lapses, however, matched the symptoms of some of the plaintiffs in various suits against Upjohn, the manufacturer of Halcion.

Millie and I had discussed the Halcion possibility once before. She argued, reasonably, that I was taking a very small dose. Only one pill. We didn't know that the effect was cumulative.

So I brought up Halcion again.

"Well," she said, "if it will make you feel better, stop taking it and let's see what happens."

I did. Within a week my problems diminished and ultimately vanished. We giggle about that now, looking back on it.

Six months later, a prominent doctor in Boston was featured on TV saying, "We've found a number of cases of false positives for neurological syphilis. Now the patients won't let us do spinal taps. It's becoming a real problem for us!"

My first working hypothesis was correct: The syphilis blood test was erroneous. But another hypothesis — that sleeping through the night was important for my health — had a little flaw in it. I assumed that FDA approval of Halcion meant it was safe to take. Even for a long time. Oops!

MANAGING STRESS AND OTHER NON-HIV HEALTH PROBLEMS

It's no surprise that people experience shingles, herpes, and other stress-related illnesses in the months after a positive HIV test. Later, after they come to terms with the information, their health improves. I've seen this repeatedly and it makes sense.

Stress causes illness even in healthy people. I reason that people with weakened immune systems are more susceptible to anything which causes illness, but *stress is particularly bad for people with HIV.*

Over the years, I've learned to manage stress in various ways. When Dr. Martinez told me I had AIDS, I asked for a Valium prescription. Valium helps me when I'm stressed. Occasionally — maybe once a month — I take a Valium before a stressful event I cannot avoid. I use it prophylactically.

A critical way to keep stress in check is to get enough sleep. During my first round of chemo, I developed insomnia. The ordeal of anticipating and then receiving an AIDS diagnosis had already made sleep difficult. Now I slept no more than a couple hours a night. I was tired, and felt lousy all the time.

Remember my Halcion tale? This is what started it. I asked Dr. Clean for a sleeping pill, to combat the insomnia. He prescribed Halcion and I slept like a log. Although I still had the other chemo side effects — constipation and minor hair loss — I felt physically much better, and more in control. Since Halcion appeared to have no side effects, I continued taking the lowest dose — one pill — nightly.

The following summer, I started taking AZT. The prescribed dose was two pills every four hours. When Bubbles told me to set my alarm and wake up at two a.m. to take pills, I said, "I think the potential benefit of those two pills in the middle of the night is outweighed by screwing up my sleep."

I knew that waking up in the middle of the night was destructive. My hypothesis was: The advantage of taking twelve pills (1200 mg) versus only ten pills (1000 mg) was questionable and probably negligible. The adverse effect of disrupting my sleep was significant and very real. I continued taking a Halcion every night for three more years, until my memory problems pushed Millie into recommending a spinal tap.

Most importantly, I manage stress and stay healthy — both mentally and physically — by being active. As a volunteer at AIDS Action, I managed difficult but rewarding projects and staff. My energy levels rose and I was invigorated.

Sometimes, however, even volunteer work can be stressful. I ultimately found this to be true at AIDS Action, when I was catapulted into a challenging job less than a year after I started volunteering.

New Year's 1989 found AIDS Action facing its first budget shortfall. Revenues were flat. By February, it was clear that layoffs would be necessary — and some reorganization. The executive director, Larry Kessler, was working full-time to increase government funding for AIDS agencies throughout New England and, increasingly, the nation. He had just been appointed to the National Commission on AIDS.

While my boss, Larry Killian, organized a financial plan, Michael Connolly was appointed personnel director and fashioned an organizational plan. Demands on AIDS Action would continue to rise, but funding would not. Therefore, internal decision making would become more difficult. To avoid logjams, a chief of operations would be needed to coordinate the department directors, a deputy executive director.

Larry Killian was not interested in this new position. He was scaling back his work, due to his recent AIDS diagnosis. The executive director, Larry Kessler, approached me. Would I become acting deputy executive director, as a volunteer, and keep the agency on track for six months while he recruited someone to work full-time?

I was flattered. It looked like a great job. Compared to my job at Yankee, where I supervised a staff of fifteen computer analysts and programmers, this position was more complex — more vital — and new. I would get to design the job!

On the other hand, the design I had in mind could be stressful. I debated with myself. Finally I said, "Would I take this job if I weren't HIV-infected?" The answer was yes. I decided to go ahead.

My first day was March 15, 1989. On the door of my new office, I found a crayon-lettered sign saying, "Deputy Bob," with a silver star pinned beneath it. My career was spiraling upwards!

By June, the balance was tipping from challenging to stressful. It was budget season. Layoffs were in process. The Three Musketeers had done their annual budgets early and fled to France for the month of May. And the fundraising direc- tor had resigned, so I was managing that department person- ally, as well as managing the other department directors. In addition, I was negotiating with my clinic for a primary care physician. I was juggling a lot of balls at once and half of them seemed to be on fire! To unwind, I began having a martini after work. This was not enough. Although I loved my work, the stress was affecting my health and my home life.

I talked to Larry Killian. He had started seeing a therapist, Andre, whom he praised as intelligent, gay, and "not too crazy." When I asked Larry about managing stress, he directed me to Andre. I was concerned enough to try.

Andre's office was organized as fastidiously as he was coiffed. I told Andre I wanted to manage the stress in my life better. After reviewing my family history and current situation with him, I asked, "What will your goals be, Andre? I don't want to lie on a couch for years talking about my feelings."

"What do you want?" he replied.

"I want it to be 1975, I'm twenty-five, and there is no AIDS."

"I'm afraid I can't do that, Bob!"

"Well then, what *can* you do?"

"We can talk about what stresses you. Then we can try out solutions."

I agreed. Over the next year, Andre taught me to recognize my own stress signs, to understand and negotiate more effectively with Mario, and to communicate better with Millie, my new primary care physician. I had to admit, he was helping me manage stress. To keep him in his place, I made a point of telling him about all the sick mental health professionals I was encountering in my new job as deputy director at AIDS Action.

Here's some of what I learned: Stress is hazardous to my health. It's critical to recognize and manage it well. When I am stressed, I have trouble sleeping, my concentration at work is poor, I'm anxious, and I fight with Mario. Things I normally enjoy, like cooking dinner, are not relaxing. I need to identify what's off and take action to fix it.

How do *you* know when you are stressed? Do you:
- get insomnia?
- sleep all the time?
- have herpes outbreaks?
- drink too much?
- have trouble concentrating?
- have sweaty palms, heart palpitations?
- eat entire boxes of donuts?
- stop eating altogether?
- have arguments with friends or lover?
- start having strange sex?
- shop till you drop?
- throw up at diplomatic dinners?

Can you identify which people or activities are causing the stress? Which items can you eliminate or reduce? Could you have a friend do your taxes for you? Could you buy an answering machine and screen your calls? Hire a maid?

Managing stress also means exercising, eating right, and relaxing just as you were supposed to before HIV. Now those things are even more important. You know what makes you feel healthier. *Do it.* If you can't remember, sit down with a therapist, friend, or doctor, and review your past history.

Before HIV, I exercised five days a week. After my diagnosis, it was a couple years before my health was stable again. Now I bicycle and rollerblade regularly.

I'm not getting holistic here. Exercise may not be what works for you. Maybe it's a martini. Fine! Listen to your body and respond. That may do as much good as any antiviral drug. I'm assuming that your body speaks reasonably to you. Mine has never told me to have twinkies and ice cream for breakfast.

For example, I go through periods when I crave salads and green vegetables. Overall, I want more carbohydrates — pasta, rice, mashed potatoes — than before HIV. Other times I really want fried food. In each case, I give my body what it wants. My friends declare me the Master of Rationalization.

SMALL RED FLAGS

I believe that HIV weakens your immune system enough that a bad cold or a severe bout of flu can trigger a more serious illness. It's a domino effect. In my case, a flare-up of my KS. As a person with HIV, you can't afford to ignore your body the way teenagers do. You must attend to your health problems while they are minor.

Experienced car owners listen for *pings* in the engine and other small changes. These are red flags. People with HIV have seven things we can monitor in an easy, matter-of-fact way. You'll stay healthier and worry less if you attend to these red flags promptly:
- skin conditions,
- mouth and throat problems,
- bowel or digestion problems,
- unusual pains,
- weight loss,
- vision problems, and
- memory, mood, or concentration problems.

Skin conditions are a chronic issue for virtually all people with HIV. Dry patches, bumps, weird welts, flaking, you name it. I have five different skin conditions for which I use five different creams. In some cases the skin doctor has diagnosed the problem — a fungus, for example. In other cases she hasn't, but we've found a way to treat it anyway.

Don't let skin problems go, for three reasons. First, the skin is your most important barrier against infection — your first line of defense, so to speak. Don't let it get out of hand. Second, skin conditions are uncomfortable. You don't need the annoyance. Third, they are *easy* to treat!

Mouth problems like canker sores, thrush, and cracks on the lips are also common for people with HIV. Sometimes they're chronic and need treatment; sometimes they go away by themselves. My one case of thrush was years ago and lasted less than a month. Check your mouth for KS lesions, too.

Weight loss — say, five or ten pounds over a few months — is not to be confused with wasting syndrome. But it means something is wrong. If you didn't have HIV, the doctors might look for thyroid problems or food allergies. Since you do have HIV, it could also be anything from stress or depression to intestinal parasites, fungus, or KS.

Changes in bowel habits or digestion may indicate a number of things. Naturally, if you ate five potato pancakes last night, you should not be alarmed at heartburn today. If the change appears to have no cause, it could indicate a problem with your other medications. AZT, ddI, and ddC can cause bowel problems. Try taking an antacid, stool softener, or bowel regulator and see if it goes away. If it doesn't, be sure your doctor investigates, because you could have infections that are HIV-related, like KS or cryptosporidiosis.

Exceptional pain means something is wrong. If you fell off your rollerblades and banged your arm, you know why your arm hurts. If you got migraines before HIV, then you'll continue to do so. That's not what I'm talking about here. But if you have a pain in your back for no apparent reason, look into it.

Changes in vision are perhaps the most critical symptoms to respond to quickly. If you have cytomegalovirus (CMV) or herpes, you may notice cloudy vision long before an opthamologist can spot the infection. These conditions are usually very treatable if caught early. You can lose your eyesight if you leave such conditions untreated.

Difficulties with memory, mood, or concentration not

caused by stress could indicate depression. People with HIV certainly have cause for depression! Check it out. Depression is treatable, either with medication or therapy or some combination.

Think of this as a checklist. You're looking for little red flags — like the *ping* in a car engine. When talking to your doctor about little things wrong with your body, remember: Start with the simplest explanations and treatments and see what happens. Don't leap to drastic conclusions. Most of your problems will be minor, manageable conditions.

Monitoring and treating these conditions daily is a drag. Try to deal with your anger about this imposition. Join a support group, see a therapist, talk to a friend, do whatever works for you. If you were a rigidly organized person before HIV, these nuisances may be particularly frustrating. Your job is to manage HIV as a chronic illness — like an unpleasant neighbor who has moved in and will not be leaving.

Don't be in denial.
Don't rationalize your little warning signs away.

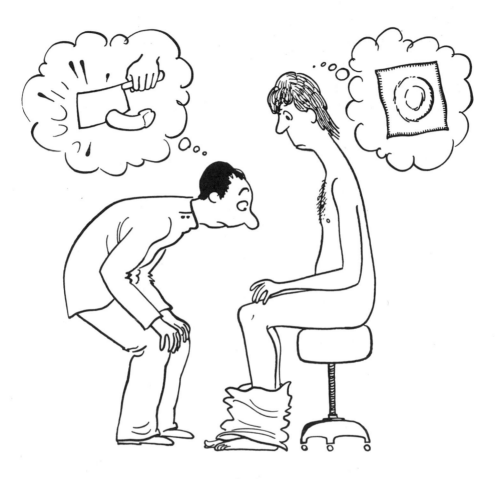

MORAL: **Treat problems empirically.**
Try simpler things first.

MONITORING YOUR HEALTH
Use this worksheet to see how these concepts might apply to you. Take this list with you when you see a new doctor.

1. List important medical conditions you had before HIV.

2. List the important HIV-related conditions you have had.

3. List the medications that disagreed with you before and after HIV.

   Before:

   After:

4. What foods disagree with you? Agree with you?

5. List the three most stressful things you have experienced in your life.

   _____

   _____

   _____

6. What are the two most stressful things going on in your life *aside from HIV?*

   _____

   _____

4

Seeking Treatment

If you want to stay alive and healthy with HIV, you must shop around for appropriate drugs and therapies. *You* are the shopper. Your doctor is your consultant. You've probably figured that out by now. That was the easy part!

The hard part is: *Neither the system nor the products operate according to simple logic.* You'll need to learn a more sophisticated logic.

1) The treatment system is not organized for shoppers.

Imagine a mall where salespeople (doctors and specialists) don't know what's available outside their own stores. New products are rumored — but no one has details. There are no glossy, up-to-date catalogs. No *Consumer Reports*. Not even a decent floor plan. The experts don't have the answers! That is the HIV treatment system. It's not like shopping for a toaster in a mall.

2) The products are unpredictable.

Drugs are not like toasters, which do the same job no matter who plugs them in. Drugs have different positive and negative effects, depending on your unique body chemistry and history. As Grace Slick sings in "White Rabbit," "One pill makes you big and one pill makes you small. The ones that mother gives you don't do anything at all." You and your doctor must make educated guesses. *No one knows for sure.*

Consequently, you have some homework to do. You must investigate treatments and assess their potential benefits and costs *as they apply to you.*

Here are some of the questions you should be asking:
- What needs to be treated?
- Do I need to treat it at this point?
- What treatments are available?
- How will I know which one will work best for me?
- What about side effects?
- Should I try experimental drugs? Which ones? At what point?
- When should I see a specialist?
- How will I know when to stop a treatment?

With information, step-by-step discussion with your practitioner, and a clear sense of your priorities, these questions can be answered.

ASSESSING COSTS AS WELL AS BENEFITS

Treatments generally have costs as well as benefits. Short-term side effects are usually well documented, but long-term costs may be overlooked.

AZT, for example, can produce a metallic taste in your mouth, headaches, nausea, and anemia. The literature describes the duration and intensity of these side effects, as well as the profile of the patient most likely to experience them. (You may not like the term "patient," but that is what we are in the literature.)

When AZT was approved for HIV treatment in 1987, the recommended dose was 1200 mg. Twelve pills a day. What were the long-term costs of pumping that much AZT through the liver every day for five years? There was no way to know precisely in 1987.

As of 1992, many practitioners are still treating HIV, and particularly AIDS, as a terminal condition. They worry about what will happen to you over the next twelve months. Sometimes, of course, this is appropriate. In any case, they're not thinking about the consequences of your drugs, radiation, or chemotherapies five or ten years out. But I am. I'm doing everything I can to ensure that I'm here in five years.

If you treat HIV as a chronic condition — something you intend to live with for a long time — you must learn to think about long-term effects. Your doctors may be assuming you'll be dead in three years — so who cares what will happen to your liver in five! But what if you think there will be a better treatment in three years and you plan to live long enough to try it out? You should be quite concerned with how much of you is left to treat!

Since there isn't much long-term data on newer treatments, you must rely on informed common sense.

I discovered this stuff as a kid. My mother ate lots of drugs. Bags of Thorazine, lithium, tryptophane, and so on. Thirty years later, her doctor found that her liver had swollen to three times its proper size. This was not the first ailment caused by her overmedication.

In my own case, sometimes the short-term situation seemed more critical, other times the long-term effects seemed more important. With AZT, I've used smaller doses. I reasoned that the harm the larger dose would do was greater than its incremental benefit. On the other hand, when I thought I was going to die real soon from KS, I let them zap me with large doses of chemotherapy and radiation. Fire away! BAM! Get that KS!

INVESTIGATING YOUR OPTIONS

Remember the story of my memory problems in chapter 3? Diagnosing the condition was a long struggle. At one point, my doctor thought the problem might be syphilis — but it turned out to be Halcion.

Let's assume you're comfortable with your diagnosis. Before you and your doctor choose between treatment options, you must do some investigating. For any treatment (pills, chemotherapy, radiation, acupuncture, whatever), you need information about four factors:

1) Efficacy
- How often does it work?
- For whom? Women or men?
- People with many T-cells or few?
- How quickly?
- How will I know?

2) Dosage
- At what dosage does it work?
- How often?
- For whom?

3) Side effects
- What are they?
- How severe?
- How frequent?
- At what dosage levels?
- For whom?
- How can they be minimized?

4) Interactions with other treatments and common medications
- Has this been studied at all?
- What data is available?
- Will taking this treatment preclude other treatments later?

Here is how I investigate options today:

1) I ask my primary care physician for an overview of the treatments.

2) I call the Gay Men's Health Crisis (GMHC) Hotline to discuss the options. GMHC sends me written information.

3) I read the information.

4) I talk with someone who is taking the treatment.

5) Then I talk to my physician again.

Treatment hotlines like those at Project Inform and GMHC (which are both listed in the appendix) are particularly helpful. They're staffed by professionals who answer treatment questions forty hours a week. They have more up-to-date information than the average doctor. Your doctor may have seen your latest problem just a few times, since HIV is one of many conditions she treats. A hotline professional at GMHC or Project Inform has probably discussed the same condition with a hundred people like you. HIV is his whole job.

This specialization can help or hinder you. "I can't sneeze without my doctor thinking it's HIV," Larry once remarked. An HIV hotline professional may do the same. He may view your symptoms as HIV-related when the condition is something else — perhaps chronic fatigue syndrome, or an allergy. Remember, hotline staff are absolutely dependent on what you remember to tell them about your situation.

No one has the gospel truth — not the doctors, the

newsletters, or the hotlines. *Make sense of what you read by talking it over with other people.* Test your understanding and logic by rephrasing what you've learned. Explain how you think the treatment might affect you, and why. Ask for feedback. Hotline professionals, in particular, have the patience and training for this. Your nurse or physician's assistant (PA) may also. Your doctor may be less forthcoming. In chapter 5 I'll discuss how to train him.

You must do your homework before discussing treatment decisions with your practitioner. Only then can you compare information and reasoning when the doctor recommends a treatment you feel uncomfortable about. If you have no information of your own, the discussion can grind to a halt — or become adversarial. You are not making good use of your practitioner's time or your own.

Showing up prepared will allow you to engage with the doctor. If you want the relationship to be a partnership, you must do your share.

DIALOGUE WITH YOUR PRACTITIONER

HIV treatments are not like hammers and nails. A simple *bang bang* won't fix everything. Medical treatments are very complex and subtle, and they work differently on different patients. You need to check out your doctor's assumptions about why a treatment would or would not work for you. The assumptions could be wrong, even if the logic is good.

There are a number of reasons why your doctor may have misinformation or faulty assumptions, not the least of which may be you. For starters, you may not have clearly communicated how you're feeling now and why it is a problem.

Assuming you have done so — and that you and your doctor are comfortable with a diagnosis — reflect on your medical history. That is Step One. The onus is on you to review your medical history with your practitioner. What about that tetanus shot in 1970 that made your face swell up and turn blue? It could be buried so deeply in your medical record that no one knows it's there. Knowing about such an incident could completely change the approach your doctor recommends.

The two of you may have different information about a given treatment. Have you shared that information? Have you asked whose facts are more current? Have you considered which source is more comprehensive? Are they equally credible? Finally, have you compared her logic and yours about why a certain drug or dosage level might work for you? These are exactly the things you need to discuss with your doctor.

I've been a poster boy for the latest mainstream treatments. When alpha-interferon, AZT, and ddI came out, I was there. As someone on top of the literature, when something new popped up, so did I.

In 1986, the big drug was interferon. I read about it during my first course of chemo. Although it wasn't approved for treatment of HIV itself, doctors were using it to treat KS. Interferon was supposed to boost your immune system and thus increase your ability to fight KS and other opportunistic infections (OIs). I wondered if it might help the body fight HIV itself, not just the KS.

At the end of 1986, my lesions began spreading again. I'd already tried chemo a few times, and I'd tried one course of radiation. The KS would go dormant for a couple months, then start up again. I told Doc Clean I wanted to look into interferon. Because interferon was new, he scheduled me to see his boss, Bubbles.

I was sitting in the Oncology waiting room when Bubbles handed me a big packet of technical materials on interferon. "This just came today," he said. "I haven't had a chance to study it yet. I have two more patients. Why don't you read it. Then you can tell me if you want to do it."

I felt good about this. Since starting chemo with Dr. Clean in June, I'd talked to Bubbles several times, whenever we ran into difficult questions. He was always willing to explain his logic and listen to mine. He engaged with me. We were developing a rapport.

There I was, studying this big stack of very technical material. Side effects, efficacy rates, charts, tables. Most of it I understood, but not all. I was doing my homework right then. Thirty minutes later, Bubbles called me into his office.

"Well, do you want to do it?"

"What's the standard dose?" I asked.

"You take a lot of this stuff. Thirty million units every other day, I think."

"What is the low dose and the high dose?"

He looked through the documents and found the dosage data. The labeling on the chart was so technical I hadn't realized it was about dosage.

"This is a chemotherapy, really," Bubbles explained. "You want a high dose to be effective."

As a trained oncologist, Bubbles's philosophy was to really zap you. At the time, I accepted that.

"When should I notice it's working?" I asked. We rifled through the documents again. That was unclear. Few of the patients studied had KS.

"What are the efficacy rates at different doses?" I asked. We checked. Patients on the high dose responded much more often than those on the standard and low doses. The graph looked something like this:

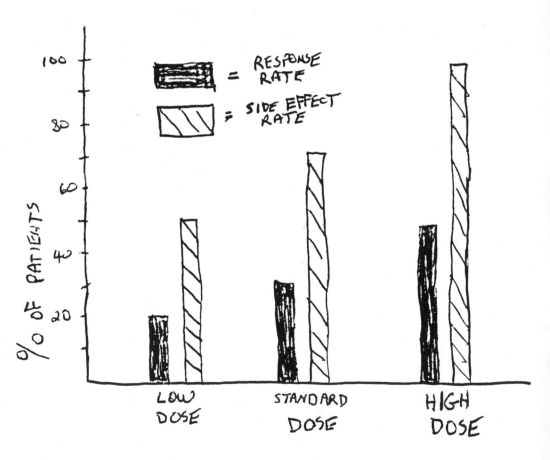

It looked promising — but there was troubling data, too. "According to this literature," I said, "the side effects depend on the dose." At standard and high doses, the side effects were common and sometimes severe.

This raised the issue of how much risk I wanted to bear. The graph showed roughly a 20 percent probability of responding to interferon at the low dose, a 30 percent probability of responding at the standard dose, and a 45 percent probability at the high dose. The data also showed a 50 percent probability of side effects at the low dose, 70 percent at the standard dose, and over 90 percent at the high dose. Bubbles recommended a high dose rather than the standard dose.

Did I want to run a 20 percent greater risk of side effects for the extra 15 percent probability that I would respond? That is what I, as the patient, had to decide.

"The side effects look bad," I said dubiously.

"I've heard they're really not that bad."

"But, Glenn, they say everyone on this gets the flu!" I flipped to an earlier page. "Look here — 98 percent of patients had severe flu symptoms at this dosage. And listen to how they define severe. 'Fevers of 102 to 104 degrees about eight hours after injection.' And fatigue, aches, and nausea. You may not consider that to be serious, but I sure as hell do!"

"It only lasts a day, Bob!"

"But I'll have to inject myself every other day!"

At the end of the session, we had still had a few questions. Bubbles agreed to make some calls to New York, where they had more experience giving interferon to people with AIDS. Hardly anyone in Boston was taking interferon in 1987.

I decided to try the interferon. I already had a dozen lesions and was worried. I wanted to waste no time.

I let Bubbles give me thirty million units every other day. That was on the high side of the standard dose. Today, the standard dose is one to three million units every other day. I was doing ten to thirty times the dose people get today.

Here is what happened.

First, it was a production just administering my injection. I have always shuddered at needles. Now I had to inject myself every other day.

I came into Oncology for training. Paula, a nurse, showed me how to fill the needle — a huge horse needle. I did that and stuck it into an orange. Then she left me for a few minutes to practice. I looked down at my leg. I thought of orange pulp and felt sick.

"Here's a week's supply of needles," said Paula when she returned. She had me stick myself. I did.

"Do you have any questions?"

I didn't. What's to ask when you are at the top of the roller coaster looking down?

The next day, I began the drama by taking half a Valium and sitting on my bed, wearing only my bathrobe. I stared at the needle and at my leg, willing it to happen. Then I stuck — and it hurt like hell. My heart sank.

That evening my sister-in-law Jean called. "Rob, there's a spirit on your porch. Right now!"

"R-e-a-l-l-y, Jean!" I replied. "What shall I do with this information?"

"I don't know. I just thought you should know. I have a bad feeling about it."

I thanked her and wondered if the bad spirit was the interferon in my refrigerator.

The next shot was no better, nor the one after that.

When I went back to Oncology the next week, I was greeted by a different nurse, Jane.

"God, this hurts!" I told her.

"How big are the needles you're using?"

I showed her with my fingers — over three inches long.

"Oh, no. There are smaller ones. Just one inch and much slimmer. They hurt a lot less."

Later, Jane taught me to inject myself in the stomach. Usually that was painless, but every fourth time or so I hit something and really yelped!

Six to eight hours later, without fail, the flu side effects would hit me like a truck. The fevers went as high as 104.

"Don't worry," Jane told me, "after a month your body will get used to it."

My fevers did drop — to a mere 101! Instead of being violently ill, I was only very sick. Sometimes I stayed the whole day in bed.

As spring began, I got weaker and weaker. Between January and May, I lost thirty pounds — 25 percent of my body weight. By Memorial Day, I was too weak to walk down the driveway to the mailbox.

Mario increasingly found himself caring for me. A first-born Italian son, he had never cooked a meal before we met — and still thought he needed a passport to get into the supermarket. As I got sicker, I criticized everything he did. I'm an independent person and my independence seemed to be disappearing altogether. No matter how much Mario did, it wasn't enough. "These vegetables aren't right. This is a lousy cut of meat." And so on.

In spite of the horror of it all, the interferon was in fact working. It stopped my KS altogether. I had no new lesions, and some old ones shrank. But after losing thirty pounds, I decided this was no longer acceptable. I was tired and miserable, and nasty to Mario. I might as well be dead. I threw the syringe at the kitchen wall one early June morning. I'd had enough. I stopped interferon.

My KS stayed under control. By late summer I felt better. My strength was back and I had gained weight. I was not sure it had been worth it, though.

Three years later, however, Jane told me she thought the massive dose of interferon was what had kept me reasonably healthy. Bubbles may have been right. I have yet to detect any negative long-term effects.

Today, doctors shift to a lower dose (called a "maintenance dose") once they achieve the primary desired effect. Some data suggests that a big initial zap works. I was willing to go with the massive dose because I thought I was terminal.

Would I make the same decision again? That depends. I would ask for data on survival rates. If there was a 40 percent chance the treatment would prolong my life significantly — say, two or three years — I would do it again. For only six months or a year? No.

The first real HIV drug was AZT, which the FDA approved a few weeks after I stopped interferon, in June 1987. When I had started interferon, AZT was still experimental. The first round of studies (called Phase One) had shown that AZT was moderately toxic, but effective. Burroughs Wellcome, the manufacturer, went on to research efficacy at different dosages (Phase Two). When the FDA approved AZT, I clipped the article. In early July, I brought it with me to an appointment with Bubbles.

"I'd like to try AZT," I said.

"I can't get it yet," he told me. "It's not really available."

When I got home, I called Project Inform in San Francisco. "How do I get AZT?"

A volunteer told me that Burroughs Wellcome had an AZT hotline. Great! I called it right away.

"Can my doctor get AZT?" I asked. "How do *I* get it?"

"That's easy," said the voice at the other end. "Your doctor can write you a prescription. Then you go to the drugstore!"

I dialed Bubbles and reached his administrative assistant. Bubbles was with a patient.

"This is important," I began. "Bubbles told me this morning that he can't get me AZT. But the drug company just said all he has to do is write a prescription!"

"Shouldn't he know that?"

"Yes, he should! Please say I need him to write a prescription today."

He did and I took it to the drugstore that afternoon. I had the pills within a week.

This is the first antiviral for AIDS, I thought, *and my doctor doesn't know he can get it.*

By early autumn, my KS was still in check — and I felt good. This was the longest period I had gone without a flare-up. Some of my old lesions were still there, though, maybe a little smaller and lighter. In October, I asked Bubbles what he thought about AZT.

"There are so many variables, it's hard to say," he replied.

"Those variables would be there if I did chemo, too. What would you call this kind of response if it occurred after chemo?"

"A partial response."

"So you're saying the AZT worked?"

"No, I can't say that."

"But if I were on chemotherapy and had this exact response you would say it worked, right?"

"Well, yeah."

A year later, Bubbles mentioned that he was treating all his KS patients with low-dose antivirals and chemo. In the long run, he thought the combination was more effective and less harmful than high-dose chemotherapy alone.

Bubbles and I have taught each other a lot over the years.

He has explained different chemotherapies and showed me how to think about the differences between chemotherapies and antivirals. He treated me as a colleague. I suggested combining a low dose of AZT with chemo, which we did. And it worked. Moreover, Bubbles acknowledged that it worked. And when he was right, he pointed that out too!

Three years later, I made an appointment with Bubbles to discuss memory problems — which turned out to be Halcion-induced. At the outset, Bubbles said he doubted he could offer any insight into my memory problems. "It sounds like dementia and that's not an oncology problem."

"Oh well," I said, "what's new with you?" Bubbles began talking about his own career. He told me that a big portion of his patient load was people with HIV, and he talked about how difficult it was to see so many patients his own age dying. "I didn't go to medical school to become an AIDS doctor," he reflected. "I wanted to be an oncologist."

"I think I know what you mean," I responded. I told him about friends and colleagues I had lost. "Of course, when I got my MBA," I added, "I didn't plan on having AIDS — or living off of disability insurance!"

When our time was up, forty-five minutes later, I realized we never got back to my memory problems. Nonetheless, I considered it time well spent. We hadn't had this kind of chat in ages. The following week, Millie told me she'd received a letter from Bubbles expressing his concern.

COMMUNICATING WHAT'S IMPORTANT TO YOU

Good treatment decisions depend not only on information, assumptions, and logic, as described in the previous section. What you treat, how you treat it, and when or if you treat it will also depend on values and priorities. What's important to *you*?

Around Christmas of 1987, I had two lesions the size of peas on my right hand. They were growing slowly, but I was concerned that they might spread. Having had a successful course of radiation therapy in 1986, I raised that possibility with Bubbles.

"Radiation is dangerous," he reminded me. "They'll only treat an area — arm, leg, whatever — twice in your life. We can't refer you to Radiation Therapy unless the lesions hurt." I let the matter drop. It was not that important yet.

In January, I was having dinner with my brother Stevie and his wife, Jean. Tommy, my three-year-old nephew, remembered the lesions from my previous visit.

"Uncle Rob. How'd you get the booboo? And why won't it go away?"

"I don't know, Tommy," I replied.

At home that night, I thought, *If my three-year-old nephew is upset about these lesions, what about my thirty-year-old friends?*

The next day I marched into Oncology and said, "These lesions are really starting to hurt." I got my referral to Radiation and we radiated ten or twelve times. The lesions faded and shrank. Although the procedure was "We treat it when it hurts," it was up to me to define "when it hurts." Thus, I decided *when* to treat based on *my* priorities.

Your priorities may also affect your choice of treatment.

Like many people with HIV, I take aerosolized pentamidine (AP) to prevent pneumocystis pneumonia (PCP). I've been taking AP monthly since 1988, because it's the recommended treatment. It seems to work — I've never had PCP. However, because I have sinus problems, inhaling the AP inflames my sinuses and my lungs. For the rest of the day, my ears hurt and I feel lousy.

There are other options — Bactrim and Dapsone, to name two. In February 1992, I considered switching to Bactrim, because recent data suggested it was more effective than AP.

Let's go back to what I said earlier about investigating your options. What does "more effective" mean?

Is Bactrim more effective for people like me who have been taking AP for four years?

Is it more effective if you've never had a bout of PCP? (I haven't.)

Or does Bactrim work better for people who have already had PCP?

What if you only have KS?

Does Bactrim's efficacy depend on how many T4 cells you have?

And if it is effective for people like me, will it improve my quality of life? Will the side effects be more acceptable than with AP?

These are the questions I was asking. Averages don't

mean that much. No one has 2.2 children. What counts is the data behind the averages. Here's what I've found so far.

Bactrim is a pill taken daily; it circulates throughout your body, and finally passes through the liver, before it is secreted out. Because it affects the whole body, it's called a *systemic* treatment. I don't much like taking pills. (Unless, of course, the side effects are fun.) Since Bactrim is taken daily and indefinitely, I was also concerned about long-term effects.

AP, on the other hand, is a *localized* treatment. You inhale it straight into your lungs, where the PCP usually hangs out. Remember, PCP is an opportunistic infection that lives in the lungs and is normally held in check by the immune system.

Shortly before my AP treatment I discussed this with Millie, my primary care physician. Millie knows I don't tolerate AP well.

"Millie," I began, "what are the side effects of Bactrim?"

"Nausea is what I've heard."

"How many people get nausea?"

"I don't know." She scanned a menu on her computer screen. "Look, we can find out."

I pulled my chair to her side and watched as she tapped on the keyboard. Information flashed on the screen.

I sighed. "Half of them report nausea!"

"It may not be that bad, Bob. They haven't said it was severe."

"True," I conceded, "but I don't want to be sick every day, even just a little." I ticked off my activities — seeing friends and family, spouse maintenance, AIDS activism, bicycling, all the household shopping, and writing this book. I need to be out and about. I get energy from being with other people, and it's a priority. (You may have different priorities. Communicate them to your doctor.)

Millie cocked her head. "You thought Bactrim would be easier than AP and now you're not sure?"

"Exactly. I'd rather be pretty sick one day a month than feel a little nauseated all the time. Or even half the time! I want to lead as normal a life as possible."

"You could try it and see," she offered.

I thought about it. "I'd rather not, unless my reaction to the AP gets worse. If you get more information about who

Bactrim works better on, let me know."

She agreed and that's how we left it. For the past year my health and daily routine had been stable and I wasn't ready to risk throwing them off kilter without more information. By coincidence, the problem resolved itself without any action on my part. At my next AP treatment, the hospital was using a new inhaler. The mist was finer and the process took half as long. For the first time in years, I felt okay after my AP treatment. There was no need to continue investigating Bactrim.

I had planned to speak with the Infectious Diseases (ID) doctors at my facility. I'm lucky. I have access to specialists who will see me or return my calls. If you can create the same kind of situation, do it. It will be helpful.

I consider my primary care physician to be just a starting point inside the medical facility — a gatekeeper, so to speak. She could talk to the Infectious Diseases doc for me, but I don't want to lose the interaction with the specialists and the opportunity to check out their assumptions.

Suppose the ID doc told Millie, "Bactrim is a better treatment. It works for everyone except people who've had lots of interferon." Millie, who might have forgotten that I had interferon in 1987 before she knew me, would come back to me and say, "Let's do it."

If I discussed the issue with the ID doctor directly, however, I could ask, "Who does it work best with? What conditions are ruled out?" and so forth. And when he said, "Well, the only population it seems to be less effective for are those who have been on interferon," I would say, "Oh, but I *have* taken interferon — lots of it." And we would consider another course of action.

How could a glitch like this happen with specialists? Think of the moving parts!

- Have you or your doctor communicated your situation effectively to the specialist?
- Has the specialist obtained your medical record?
- Has she read only the first page or read the whole record?
- Was your information recorded correctly?
- Was all the information put in there to begin with?
- Does your specialist remember what she read in your record?

- Maybe she attended the office Christmas party last night?
- Maybe you attended a party last night?

And so on.

Then, of course, there is the issue we raised in chapter 1: You may know more than the doctor. You may not. You'll never know for sure unless you ask questions.

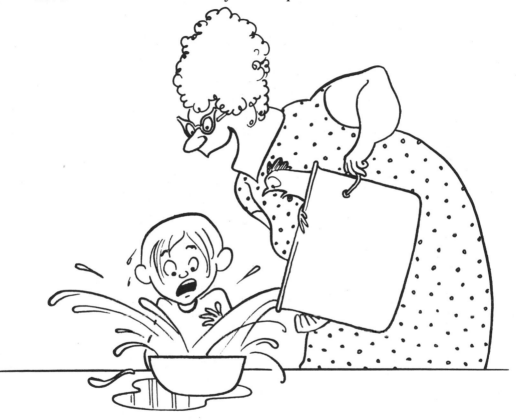

MORAL: **More medicine is not always better.**

Treat HIV as a chronic condition, rather than as a terminal one.

SEEKING TREATMENT
Use this worksheet to see how these concepts might apply to you.

1. List occasions before HIV when you or a family member were not treated optimally by a doctor.

2 Can you name any FDA-approved drugs that have caused more harm than good? List them here.

3. What condition are you considering treatment for now?

4. From which of the following have you requested written information?

_____ GMHC Treatment News

_____ Project Inform

_____ Your local Body Positive chapter

_____ Your local ACT-UP chapter

_____ Positive Direction's newsletter

_____ Your local AIDS service organization

_____ Your nurse or doctor

_____ Your local public health department

5. What treatments are you considering?

6. What questions do you need to ask your doctor?

What is the efficacy of this treatment? How often does it work?

For which patients does it work?

How often does it work at the different doses?

How will we know it is working?

At what doses are there side effects?

How frequent are the side effects at different doses?

How severe are the side effects at different doses?

7. What quality of life issues are important to you today? What kind of side effects are not acceptable? Why?

5

Managing
Your Doctor

P eople want to assume that all doctors are good. That assumption may kill you.

If you still think all doctors are brilliant, well informed about HIV infection, and solely interested in your well-being, and if you like following their recommendations blindly, then skip this chapter. If you assume all doctors are incompetent, ill-informed, and unethical, you should see a therapist. Doctors are just like other professionals. Most are adequate, but some are very good and some are very bad. You must evaluate them individually and determine if they fit your needs.

Here are some questions you should be asking:

- What do I need from a primary care physician?
- What should I realistically expect?
- How important is a good medical facility?
- How do I communicate what I need to my doctor?
- How can I tell if I have a good doctor?
- How can I tell if she's doing a good job?
- What do I do if she doesn't have all the information I need?
- What should I do if she's not doing what I want?
- How do I find a new doctor?

In this chapter, I'll show you how to choose an appropriate doctor, communicate expectations effectively, and get good service.

KNOWING WHAT YOU WANT: THE JOB DESCRIPTION

George is a successful photographer living on the Upper West Side of Manhattan. In 1986, he had a bout of shingles.

At the time, George had no doctor. Knowing that shingles is an early symptom of HIV infection, George got an anonymous HIV test, which came back positive. Next, he sought out a noted infectious disease doctor, Scott Jenkins, who had treated hundreds of HIV patients since 1983.

Jenkins did an extensive blood screening, with the exception of a T4 test, which he said should be kept off the record. For that, Jenkins sent George to a New York hospital under the name of Benjamin Adams. "Benjamin" took the T4 test and paid for it with cash because, of course, the fictitious Benjamin Adams had no insurance. Meanwhile, Jenkins billed the "normal" blood tests to George's insurance company.

Since then, Jenkins has continued to monitor George's health, conducting normal blood tests in his office and sending George out for "anonymous" T4 cell tests.

Recently George's T4 count dropped to 550 — half the normal count. "I was terrified," he recounted to me over the phone. "When Scott told me my T4 count was dropping, we both cried. He held me in his arms and I felt safe."

Scott then wrote him a prescription for 300 mg of AZT daily. George started taking AZT, but he had doubts about it. He had heard that AZT destroyed bone marrow cells and he knew many HIV-infected people who practiced alternative therapies. The night before an appointment with Scott, he called to tell me he planned to stop seeing Scott and look for an expert in herbal therapies.

Some of the questions I asked were:

How quickly have your T-cells been dropping?

Is Scott willing to let you supplement your AZT treatment with alternative therapies?

If you feel safe with Scott, why not discuss alternative therapies with him first?

I reminded George that I had taken 1200 mg of AZT daily — four times his dose — concurrently with chemotherapy and suffered no bone marrow problems. With his T-cells at 550, it was unlikely that he would suffer bone marrow damage.

"Moreover," I said, "if AZT causes problems, you can always stop. The damage will probably reverse itself. My doctor tells her patients they can try alternative therapies, but to continue mainstream treatment. And she asks that they keep the dosage of the alternative therapy small enough that no harm is done. Why don't you ask Scott what he thinks?"

The next day, George brought these issues to Scott, who said he knew little about alternative therapies but would look into it. "Assuming there's nothing negative in the literature, I have no problem with you doing both AZT and herbs."

George called me back, much calmer. I explained that if I had found a primary care physician like Scott early in my treatment, my outlook on the medical system might be quite different. George and Scott were partners.

As it was, it took three years until I realized, in 1989:

**_Primary care physicians aren't really doctors —_
they're medical coordinators.**

Here's what happened.

My first primary care physician, Dr. Martinez, was a resident. When I was undergoing my initial course of chemotherapy in 1986, Martinez left Beth Israel. I was surprised and angry to learn that this was routine; residents stay only a year at teaching hospitals. This turnover creates problems. Even an enlightened patient doesn't have time to build rapport and train a doctor in a year.

A couple of years later, I was assigned another primary care physician, also a resident. Let's call him Harry. I could reach Harry only by going through the switchboard at Health Care Associates, the outpatient clinic I use at Beth Israel. This was just impossible. The switchboard itself was usually busy. When I got through, Harry was never available; he rarely returned my calls, even when the problem was relatively serious. After a while I just didn't bother.

Instead, I saw my oncologist, Bubbles, whom I liked. By treating my earaches and other minor problems, he allowed me to do without a primary care physician.

In spring of 1989, however, a drama began which changed all that. The lesions on my legs, torso, and arms began spreading, slowly at first, then more rapidly. AZT was no longer working. I knew my internal lesions must be spreading, too. Soon it would be a life-and-death scenario.

Meanwhile, the doctors gave me contradictory advice. Oncology wanted to try chemo again. Radiation Therapy recommended another course of radiation. And the Infectious

Disease docs wanted to increase my dose of AZT. They didn't believe it had stopped working and were ambivalent about trying anything new.

Each specialist thought the appropriate treatment lay in his area of expertise. Everyone had an opinion — and I had serious reservations about each. I had undergone numerous courses of chemotherapy and radiation. Those options get riskier and less effective with each repetition. At the rate my illness was progressing, time was of the essence. I might not get a second chance if I made the wrong choice.

I tried unsuccessfully to get the specialists to meet and discuss the pros and cons of each treatment. Hah! No one wanted to. That's not the procedure.

AZT had stopped working. Although the doctors wouldn't admit they could tell when AZT stopped working, most PWAs knew it happened between 12 and 24 months. I could certainly feel it. I'd been taking AZT for 20 months and was now losing weight. My T4s were dropping and the KS was out of control. I needed something else — and soon.

Since I had not only tolerated but responded well to AZT, I thought I would do well on another antiviral. Of the various possibilities, ddI was further along in clinical trials and looked promising. It became my drug of choice. As an experimental drug, ddI was still difficult to get from the manufacturer, Bristol-Myers. I had chosen them, but they had not yet chosen me.

I had already spoken to a few people at Beth Israel. Now I lined up additional appointments with the Infectious Disease chain of command. At this point, I received a form letter from Harry, saying, "It's been a pleasure serving you. Please contact Health Care Associates to arrange another primary care physician. Good-bye!"

Earlier, I would have taken little notice of Harry's departure and continued seeing Oncology. But the Oncology department's AIDS caseload was growing and they wanted me to get a primary care physician. Moreover, like most hospitals, Beth Israel required that you go through a primary care physician when seeking experimental drugs — a course of action I was now considering. Harry's departure became an opportunity.

For the first time, I consciously set out to hire a

primary care physician. This was a challenge I had avoided because it was bound to be time-consuming and most likely disappointing. I had hoped primary care physicians could be superdoctors and maybe colleagues, but I found they had tendencies I would never tolerate in a colleague. They were short on knowledge and long on control.

I began thinking about how a primary care physician might help me. What should I expect? Could I get a primary care physician who would coordinate the specialists and help me analyze their conflicting opinions?

Here's the job description I developed:

POSITION: Primary Care Physician,
a.k.a. Bob's Medical Services Coordinator

Duties:
- be reachable and return phone calls promptly
- write letters to disability insurance and SSI
- make referrals to specialists and iron out snafus
- help me assess conflicting opinions given by specialists
- give me my flu shots
- write prescriptions
- help me get new drugs

Qualifications:
- Previous HIV experience
- Good education
- Administrative skills or potential
- Continuity (plans to stay for a while)
- Not prejudiced
- Personable

You may think there's not much about being a "serious doctor" here. It's an administrative description. But it's also very health-related and anything but routine.

For example, when a specialist says he can't see you for three months even though your need is critical, you need someone to make the system work. Even minor snafus can cause major hassles. Bubbles often omitted the Drug Enforcement Agency (DEA) number on my painkiller prescriptions, in 1986. I'd get to the drugstore and have to go back and get the prescription fixed. If it wasn't one error it was another. Bubbles was a smart man but a terrible administrator, and that deficiency took a toll on my health.

Finally, nonmedical administrative matters have health consequences. Imagine for a moment what would happen if my disability payments were interrupted. Think of the stress.

The most important thing I figured out was: *You don't get complex medical information from your primary care physician. You get it from the specialists:* the eye doctor, oncologist, radiation therapist, respiratory care doc, infectious disease person, internal medicine doctor, dermatologist, and so on. When you get sick, you are sent to one of these people. Or several.

No primary care physician could possibly play all those roles. But she might be able to help you navigate the bureaucracy. Furthermore, if she's at a good medical facility, you get one-stop shopping. If one specialist doesn't quite fit the bill, you can go on to the next.

As I reflected on my experiences with Dr. Martinez, Dr. Clean, and Bubbles, I formulated general qualifications. First, I needed someone with experience in HIV disease. My situation was advanced and precarious. There was no getting around the fact that I was a guinea pig in the medical system. I couldn't accept a novice handler. Second, I wanted someone with a reasonably small ego. There needed to be room in the relationship for both of us. Finally, as a gay man with AIDS, I needed a nonhomophobic doctor. My experience had been that straight men don't work. The underlying homophobia gets in the way.

Here's one story about that. When Dr. Clean was reviewing my progress on chemotherapy, I shared what I thought was good news: I was feeling better and I had my sex drive back. I read the look he gave me: "That's just what society needs. Another homo who has his sex drive back. With AIDS, no less!" He was horrified that I was talking about sex at all. He was so horrified that he didn't hear what I was communicating to him — that I was feeling well — *that the treatment was working.*

What would he have preferred? That I censor my wellness reports?

Clean had deficiencies as a specialist. At the time, I thought I could find no one better, so I tolerated them. These deficiencies would have been intolerable in a primary care physician, however.

Hiring a doctor is like hiring a plumber. If you want to fix a faucet you don't obsess about what kind of a plumber you get; if you're putting in copper piping, you're much pickier. With doctors it's the same. If you need a flu shot, anyone will do. But HIV-related infections are different. They're complicated. Sort of like an old house that needs new plumbing.

First, HIV-related infections are numerous and diverse. Some are quite rare and poorly understood. Each one must be treated differently and they interact in unknown, complex ways. Second, knowledge about HIV and its treatment is constantly changing. The number of experimental therapies is bewildering. Finally, there are complex legal, economic, and governmental aspects to HIV. It's not like diabetes. People with diabetes don't worry about being thrown out of their homes, or getting mugged in the streets — or done in by their insurance company.

In sum, a person with HIV is dealing with five moving targets:

- the virus,
- the available treatments,
- his body's responses to both the virus and the treatments,
- his doctor's current knowledge or lack thereof, and
- society's current level of HIV phobia.

It's complicated.

To stay on top of new treatments, you must gather information constantly. When you find something promising, you need help navigating the system. This is where system-sense comes in. Just knowing your destination isn't enough. There are dead ends and bear traps along the way. You must be willing to take odd routes. And sometimes you'll need the help of insiders.

Medical bureaucracies, like many others, are drowning in information, choking on it, and barfing it up. I needed help analyzing the information and, once I'd made a treatment choice, working the system. Doing this alone is too stressful — even for me. And it's clearly not the realm of the specialists. I wanted a primary care physician who understood this. More importantly, I wanted someone who understood that ultimately *I made the choices.*

You may still be thinking it's bold to have requirements for your primary care physician. It's not. Think of times you needed an assistant, a colleague, a boss ... or even a boyfriend. In each case, you had requirements. The trick is first to define them, then to get comfortable discussing them. Let's turn to that next.

INTERVIEWING THE APPLICANTS

After developing the job description, I called the receptionist at Health Care Associates. He processed all requests for primary care physicians. That tells you how much importance my clinic put on matching doctors and patients. It was completely perfunctory.

Given the complexity and urgency of my situation, I explained that I needed someone experienced in HIV disease. He gave me an appointment — four weeks down the road — with a doctor I'll call Cornfield. (Position posted. First candidate.)

Dr. Cornfield turned out to be a student — a resident, I guess — from Kansas. A nice kid who spoke carefully and slowly. New to Boston. I could see he was a bit intimidated by the city and the hospital, so I tried to set him at ease by chatting about where he'd gone to school and what it was like to move to Boston. And I got him to admit that I was the first PWA he'd ever met. (Probably the first homosexual, too, I thought to myself.)

"Have you ever seen a KS lesion before?" I asked.

"No," he said shyly, "but I would like to."

As Cornfield put on rubber gloves, I showed him my lesions and reviewed some events of the past months — interferon, radiation, and so forth. I didn't bother discussing ddI, because I had concluded he was hopelessly over his head.

He saw that too, and shifted a bit in his chair. "You know," he said thoughtfully, "I have to make a decision about whether, given your condition, I should treat you."

"Doctor," I said, leaning forward, "don't worry! I won't *let* you treat me. I need someone with experience." I drew myself up to my full five-feet-four and continued, "I've been trying to get a physician for months here. I told them my requirements and I got *you!* And I'm not paying for this visit, either!"

All the blood drained from Cornfield's face and he went off to speak with his supervisor. I sat there exasperated at my predicament and miserable because I'd hurt Cornfield's feelings. A few moments later, he returned and said, "Speak to the receptionist. We have another doctor in mind." I left, wordlessly.

The receptionist gave me an appointment with Marcia, who "according to the computer" was in the process of moving north from Long Island.

Before we continue, let's compare Dr. Cornfield with Dr. Jenkins (my friend George's doctor). See the chart I've done on the next page.

You might think it isn't fair to compare a 25-year-old resident to an experienced doctor. But this process provides an accurate comparison of their respective abilities to treat a gay man with HIV infection.

In 1989, I had never heard of a primary care physician like Scott Jenkins — and I doubt there are many like him. I was looking for someone whose qualifications fell between Jenkins's and Cornfield's. For my part, I wanted to investigate, analyze, and discuss medical information with my doctor. You must decide which qualifications are important for you, based on your own strengths and weaknesses.

Next month, August, brought my meeting with Marcia. Among friends, I affectionately refer to her as Millie. As I parked in the hospital lot, I found myself thinking back to Cornfield. I was still angry. My health problems were complicated; getting a novice made me furious. This was life and death, after all. We weren't dealing with a wart here.

When I got to the clinic the receptionist looked at his computer, blinked, and said, "You don't have an appointment today."

I searched for my appointment card. "But you wrote out my card yourself when you scheduled me last month!" I showed him the card, which was in his handwriting.

"You must be mistaken," he repeated coolly, and went back to his business. I began to seethe.

"Where's the supervisor?" I said loudly. "I have an appointment and this person won't help me."

A young man peered out of an office, then vanished. Then a young, professional-looking woman appeared. It was Millie.

	JENKINS	CORNFIELD
EXPERIENCE	43 years old; Infectious Disease doc specializing in HIV; had treated over 500 HIV-positive patients	25 years old; I was the first PWA he had met
HOMOPHOBIA & ATTITUDES ABOUT SEX	Gay man... discussed safer sex	Appeared asexual ... perhaps a virgin
CONTINUITY	Private practice out of the same office since 1983; no changes planned	First week at Beth Israel; would leave in a year.
AIDSPHOBIA	Had made a career of treating HIV+ people	Put on a glove before touching the KS lesion on my leg
SYSTEM-SENSE	Arranged anonymous T4 test and explained necessity of anonymity	We didn't get this far
INTERPERSONAL SKILLS	Very engaging... held George in his arms and made him feel safe	Hadn't had this training yet
PERSPECTIVE	Lived in Manhattan	Had never been to New York (I asked)

"I can see him now," she told the receptionist and beckoned me to an office. Then she excused herself. When she returned, she said, "I cannot have them screwing up my appointments."

"Well, you see how they are," I responded, showing her

the appointment card and thinking to myself, *This might work.*

"What brings you here today?" she began.

"Well, I have AIDS."

"Yes, I know that."

"I wanted to get acquainted, since you're going to be my primary care physician and I have a lot going on right now."

I assumed she had heard about me and was prepared for a difficult PWA. I, on the other hand, knew nothing about her. I could see she was five-feet-one, light brown hair, thirtyish, and well tanned. She's well tanned every summer.

I proceeded to ask her a series of questions.

Have you treated PWAs before? (Yes)

How many? (A dozen)

Where did you go to school? (The name she gave sounded like a good school)

I was trying to keep it low-key and conversational. At a certain point, Millie paused and said, "This sounds like an interview!"

I shrugged. "I just have a few concerns I want to share with you," I said, glancing casually at my agenda, where the first item read: Interview. *Doctors aren't used to being interviewed,* I thought to myself.

Millie got what I was doing. She didn't like it, but she wasn't taken aback like other doctors and she didn't act condescending.

"I'm wondering how long you'll be here," I continued. "Will you be leaving next July?"

"No," she said, "I'm planning to be here for several years."

We continued. She asked what bothered me most at Beth Israel.

"Not being able to get through to the doctors," I told her.

She offered me her page number, which I've used ever since to get my blood test results. That's a good example of her administrative strengths and weaknesses. For several months, I paged Millie to get test results. Eventually, I suggested she leave a message about the results on my home machine, so I wouldn't have to interrupt her. And that's what we do now. The page number is for serious problems, not details.

I also asked if she used computers and she said yes.

Why, you may wonder, would I want my doctor to use

computers? Well, would you ask a prospective administrative assistant if he had computer skills? Of course you would! In this case, using computers was vital if Millie was going to manage administrative details like blood tests, feedback from specialists, and letters and applications.

The computer has medical uses, too. For example, Millie can generate a chart of my T4 cell trend in just a few seconds. And she does. Recently, my liver function was elevated. I said I wanted to see the numbers plotted over time. And she did it.

So there we were. Millie met my five requirements. She had previous experience treating people with HIV. Her education sounded good. She was planning to stay at BI for a while. She had some administrative potential. And I picked up no homophobia at all.

Millie had passed the interview! I considered her hired — and on probation.

This is not to say that she was perfect. She looked at my lesions and took some blood. As we chatted, I realized she would need training. She had that typical look, the one that says, "Oh, you're gonna die; I'm not putting much energy into this. I'm not going to bother."

People with AIDS pick up on that with every doctor we meet. We got it in 1987 and we still do. In their minds, we had one drug then: AZT. When we were done with AZT, we were *done*. Time to die. Earlier, of course, PWAs had nothing. At that time it was simply, "We can't do anything for you. Have some painkillers. Have a *lot* of painkillers. See how I'm helping you?!"

So I recognized that look in her eyes. It was nothing new. It's part of a pattern.

The pattern is this: You need a drug two years before it's been approved or before the doctors realize they can get it. And so you have to get it yourself. Remember their training. The Hippocratic oath stresses, "Do no harm." Doctors fear that experimental treatments will do more harm than good until the FDA says otherwise. Most doctors aren't truly proactive.

In truth, I still haven't trained Millie to be proactive. But that's my job as the patient: to be proactive, to manage. As for me — well, Millie didn't get me right away. She'd been warned about me, but didn't know quite what to expect, as we sniffed each other over.

As I'll explain later, Millie had some performance problems, which took me nine or ten months to correct. But here we are, three years later, and she realizes I was right. If I had listened to her I would have died. Now there's a level of respect between us; it goes both ways. We respect and trust each other. I feel that she would do almost anything to help. It took a long time to develop this rapport. And now you see why continuity is so important to me.

To help you devise your own interview questions, try filling out the Requirements Worksheet that follows. For your amusement, I've also attached some supplementary interview questions. Feel free to write your own; perhaps you need a doctor who relates well to women, or to IV drug users.

Don't be afraid to ask some of these questions. If you feel shaky, bring a friend with you. The two of you can share questions. Remember, as the interviewer, your job is to *listen*. You'll be surprised at what you learn.

PRIMARY CARE PHYSICIAN SHOPPING LIST
Fill in the blanks ... or circle as appropriate, or cross out, if you don't care

TYPE OF QUALIFICATION   **YOUR REQUIREMENT**

1) EXPERIENCE

    a) Years in practice: ____ years

    b) HIV experience: Has treated ____ patients with HIV

    c) Age: ____ years old

    d) Specialty: Primary care
                              Infectious disease
                              other

2) CONTINUITY

    a) Time at this job: ____ years

    b) Plans for future: Plans on remaining
                              ____ years

3) ACCESSIBILITY

    a) How easy to reach   Has beeper
       by phone: Has voicemail
                              Promises to return phone calls within ____ hours
                              Will not make commitment

    b) How long to get an appt.

        If urgent...   ____ hours/days

        If not urgent...   ____ days/weeks

4) INTERPERSONAL SKILLS

a) Willingness to engage about medical information — Like pulling teeth -or- Offers information freely

b) Willingness to engage about personal issues — Like pulling teeth -or- Is easy to talk to

5) PREJUDICE POTENTIAL (DIFFICULTY HANDLING DIFFERENCES)

a) Same sex — Yes No Not important to me

b) Same sexual orientation — Yes No Not important to me

c) Similar background — Yes No Not important to me

d) Similar interests — Yes No Not important to me

e) Similar belief systems — Yes No Not important to me

6) ADMINISTRATIVE SKILLS

a) Verbal communication — Good Not so good

b) Written communication — Good Not so good

c) Computer literacy — Good Not so good

7) OTHER

_____   _____

_____   _____

_____   _____

_____   _____

_____   _____

Take this list with you when shopping for a doctor.

HIRING YOUR DOCTOR
Supplementary Interview Questions

Directions: Review the job description and qualifications before the interview. Try first to set the doctor at ease by asking a few friendly questions, such as "Are you new to Boston?" Once you have reviewed your basic expectations with the doctor, work your way down this list as far as you dare.

So, have you had your vacation yet? Where'd you go? Manhattan? Vegas?

Do you use computers?

Do you treat HIV as a terminal illness or as a chronic illness?

Did you know the Centers for Disease Control (CDC) says that it's impossible for HIV-infected people to have safe sex? Waddaya think about that?

Did you know that 25 percent of first-year Harvard medical students don't believe they have an ethical obligation to treat HIV-positive people? Waddaya think about that?

Would you lie to help me get an experimental drug that could save my life?

Do you think homosexuality is caused by a gland that's too small? Is it treatable?

Do you think anal intercourse should hurt? How much?

Do you think all doctors have big egos?

[Are you wondering how to estimate the size of your doctor's ego? See the next page!]

MEDICAL EGO ASSESSOR!

Directions: Rate your doctor against each item below, assigning points as indicated. Then total the points.

Add one point if your doctor...
___ Insists you call him "Doctor." Affects to have no first name.
___ Looks startled when questioned.
___ Is a straight male or tries to look like one.
___ Says, "I'm the doctor."
___ Uses the phrase "In my best medical judgment."
___ Uses words like "edema" instead of "bruise" (i.e., is hard to follow).
___ Uses the word *"procedure."*

Add two points if your doctor...
___ Reprimands you for asking questions about her logic.
___ Refers to self in third person.
___ Reminds you of Ralph Cramden.

Subtract one point if your doctor...
___ Apologizes when he is over five minutes late for an appointment.
___ Is willing to take out the *Physician's Desk Reference (PDR)* and look up information in front of you.
___ Says things like, "I didn't understand your question. Could you explain it again?"

TOTAL: ____

Interpreting your doctor's score
-3 – 0: Rabbit. Check your math. You probably made a mistake. No doctor has an ego that small.
0 – 2: Human. Approachable; hire this one!
3 – 4: Walrus. May be trainable.
5 – 6: Superhero. There's not enough room for both of you in the hospital.
7 – 8: Big as the sun. Danger! Exposure is bad for your health!

COMMUNICATING EXPECTATIONS

Once you decide your doctor fits the bill, start communicating your expectations. Begin this process during the interview. This worked with Millie.

I wanted Millie to understand that I take my health seriously and expect to be taken seriously myself. I brought an agenda — and I placed it on top of my daytimer, right in front of us, as we began. I think that surprised her.

Everyone should have an agenda when visiting the doctor, with questions listed. Doctors answer some questions and say they'll get back to you on the others, but they rarely do. Therefore, *you* must keep track. At the next appointment, you must say, "Well, what's the answer?" If you write your questions down, you'll be able to remember to ask them — and to follow up.

Here is my agenda as scribbled in my daytimer that August day in 1989:

AGENDA

1. Interview
2. Recommendations of Oncology, Radiation, and Infectious Disease
3. Application process for ddI

Things had gone reasonably well during our interview, so I mentally hired Millie and placed her on probation. Agenda Item #1 completed. Moving on, I gave her some small but important assignments as a test of her administrative and analytical abilities:

1) Speak with the doctors in Oncology, Radiology, and Infectious Disease and get their opinions;

2) Analyze their information and give me her own opinion; and

3) Get the ddI application materials from Bristol-Myers.

As I noted earlier, I was getting conflicting recommendations from different departments. Since I couldn't get the specialists to talk to each other, I needed Millie to help me analyze their assumptions, their facts, and their objectives.

This I knew: One of the Radiation Department's objectives was to persuade patients to do radiation. It's a profit center and it makes more money by enrolling more customers, so to speak. (Have you ever noticed how Radiation has better furniture and carpets and is a lot better staffed? Think about it.)

Now, the primary objective of the individual radiation therapists is indeed to treat you, but they're likely to recommend radiation because it's their line of business. They understand radiation therapy; it's the lens through which they examine problems. When you go to an oncologist for chemotherapy, you find the same pattern. In a teaching hospital, doctors have an additional objective: developing knowledge inside their discipline. They're looking for interesting "subjects" to treat.

To this day, Millie doesn't do that well on the analysis. She reports what the specialists say and adds a few superficial observations, but she's passive. No real value added. I'm partly at fault because she assumes that I know more about the subtleties of my own body than she does. So she doesn't bother; she delegates the task back to me.

Millie's final assignment was to get the paperwork to apply for ddI on what's called a "compassionate-use basis." Compassionate-use basis means you don't qualify as a good test subject, but you are in desperate straits and might benefit from the drug.

Unfortunately, we had just met and had not established a working relationship. Millie was not eager to do this. Moreover, my request conflicted with her style. Some doctors will be creative; they'll be aggressive, even lie. That's not Millie. Millie follows the rules. Her credo is: "You're not supposed to go against *procedures.*" I started to pick up on it when I asked her to get the ddI paperwork.

"But you don't qualify!" she objected.

Actually, Millie didn't know how to make me qualify. But unknown to her, however, I had used the time between my appointment with Cornfield and her arrival to obtain most of this information from a friend at the state Department of Public Health, in case Millie couldn't or wouldn't. In any event, she finally agreed to order the application materials, if only to humor me. And that was how our opening meeting concluded.

I'd asked my interview questions and gotten the information I needed to make a hiring decision. (Yes!) I had written a list of Action Items that Millie had agreed to. (Of course, I didn't *call* them "Action Items.") And I had begun communicating my expectations about how we would work together, how frankly we would talk, what she would do.

Over the next week I read the information I'd recently received on ddI. It looked like it would be difficult to qualify even for compassionate use. I studied the criteria carefully, as I will recount in the next chapter.

Eager to get going, I arrived for my second appointment with Millie, new agenda in hand. I expected her to be toting a two-inch stack of documents, including the inclusion and exclusion criteria, a description of the application process, the forms, and so on.

When I asked if she had obtained the ddI information, she said, "Oh yes, it came, but I forgot to bring it with me." She suggested that I wait until our next monthly visit. Thirty more days when I'm dying!

This goes back to the attitude I characterize as, "This isn't going to do any good. Why bother?" Millie had simply forgotten. It wasn't important to her. In my view, however, getting ddI was the only thing that could save my life at this point. It was the only thing that would do any good.

"Well, where is it?" I responded, somewhat exasperated.

"Back in my office," she replied.

"I'll wait while you get it," I said simply.

Millie looked at me and didn't know what to say. She knew I was capable of making a scene. I'd made a scene with Cornfield and something tells me she'd heard about it. It was clear she had to go get the packet. She knew she should have had it.

She ambled out and returned ten minutes later carrying the huge unopened packet, still wrapped in plastic.

"Oh, this is a lot of material," she said dubiously, "I guess I'll have to read through it."

I leaned forward and said, "Why don't we take off the plastic together?" And we did.

Since I had already studied the inclusion and exclusion criteria, I was prepared. As we scanned the material together, I pointed to a section that said I could qualify to get the drug on a compassionate-use basis if I were not responding to AZT. Bristol-Myers had included a detailed list of what constituted "not responding." I already knew I did not fit the description, but I wanted to see what Millie would say first.

Mind you, my legs were about falling off, due to KS. Unfortunately, recurrence of KS was not on the list. The indicators were:

- a T4 cell count below 50; or
- three opportunistic infections within three months; or
- weight loss of eight pounds or more in thirty days.

You really had to be dead to get ddI. This is ironic, since ddI probably works better if taken earlier, when you're healthier. That's certainly true of AZT.

"I don't see how you qualify," sighed Millie, as we read over the list. "You don't meet any of these criteria."

Be creative, Millie! I thought.

"Why not just say I do?" I offered.

"Oh, I couldn't do that," Millie responded seriously.

"Why not?"

"I could lose my license."

I had anticipated this, so I wasn't too disappointed. In retrospect, I appreciate Millie's frankness. She was describing the system to me and her part in it. Today, Millie has more experience and we have a rapport. She would be more creative and show more initiative.

Since I had already decided to go for the weight loss angle, I mentioned to Millie that I'd been losing weight recently and then said, "Why don't we check my weight again in a week instead of waiting a month for my next appointment?"

She consented, then sent me to the lab for some of the required bloodwork. Over the next week, I intentionally lost the required weight and thus we got over that little barrier.

The following week, Millie squinted at the results of blood tests. As I've said earlier, the history of bloodwork at BI is not very good. I've experienced a 10 to 20 percent error rate.

"Your uric acid reading is a little high," she said. "It falls outside the criteria listed here." She wanted to stop the process.

"This is just one detail out of dozens required," I groaned. "Just lie!"

"I can't," she responded.

I insisted I take the test again. It came out about the same and I had her submit the paperwork anyway. It was only one number out of thirty, after all!

A week later, I called from my office at AIDS Action. I wanted to see if everything was ready for submission. Millie told me one of the thirty blood tests was missing.

"Could you come over and redo the test?"

I couldn't believe it. She was going to make me go to the lab, then wait a few more days until the lab gave us a number that might not even be correct?

I lost it at that point.

"Just make up the fucking number!" I shouted into the phone. "Submit the paperwork! I'll take the test the next time I'm in. And when the results come back, call Bristol-Myers and say you made a mistake!" I slammed down the phone, quivering with frustration.

Kenneth Ann, AIDS Action's normally unflappable phone coordinator, walked up to me, eyes wide. "Who were you talking to that way?"

"My doctor!" I growled. He gasped and retreated. I was too angry to speak.

Millie almost did as I said. She used a number from a previous test and submitted the paperwork. As it turned out, when the new test results came back, it was the same number she had used.

A few weeks later, I received the ddI. My T4 count was 160 at the time. A month later it was 260. My T4s climbed up to 400 quickly and have been bouncing between 300 and 400 ever since. That's the big picture. Fast forward, as it were.

Shortly after I started the ddI, Millie and I had a particularly interesting tussle. I asked if it might ever be a good idea to take both AZT and ddI simultaneously. Mind you, at the time, Bristol-Myers required that you *cease* taking AZT when starting ddI. I had a year's supply of AZT at home and Millie knew that.

How would she feel if I took both?

She gasped a little and said, "That could be *very* dangerous."

I was skeptical. "What makes you think so?"

"No one's done it!"

"Well, do you think scientists have ever mixed them together in a test tube?"

"I don't know."

Actually, I thought, *you don't know much about the subject and you don't have to. I'm not asking you a medical question, I'm asking you a system question.* I continued, "Would you be obligated to tell Bristol-Myers if you knew I was also taking AZT?"

"Well," mused Millie, "if you *told* me I would have to tell them."

Aha! We're on the right wavelength now.

"That's interesting. What if I hadn't told you I was taking AZT, but you could determine it by a blood test? *Then* would you have to tell them?"

I had recently learned that the MCV blood test showed elevated results for people taking AZT. I reminded her of this test.

"No," she said carefully, "in that case I would suspect you were taking AZT, but I wouldn't really know."

"Well," I concluded, "if I were combining AZT and ddI treatments, I would want you to know, so you wouldn't misinterpret possible changes in my health — say, anemia. But obviously I couldn't tell you, since Bristol-Myers might cut off my ddI."

In this way I alerted her that I might take AZT and suggested she monitor my blood accordingly. In fact, I never did take AZT again. Today, lots of people take both ddI and AZT. I haven't had to. But I thought I might need to someday, if ddI wasn't working well enough. And that was not a simple medical decision between me and my doctor. The Bristol-Myers bureaucracy was now involved.

The point is that you, the patient, *must* plan carefully for all sorts of possibilities or you get in trouble. For example, at this time PWAs were not eligible to receive ddI if they were already undergoing chemotherapy. However, people already receiving ddI *were* allowed to commence chemo! Therefore, if you were investigating both chemo and ddI, it was imperative that you put the chemo on hold and get ddI first.

These rules and procedures can critically impact your health. And the doctors have not been trained to help you think them through. It's up to you to communicate your expectations in this area clearly and consistently. My expectations — hopes, really — were that Millie would alert me to administrative procedures that threaten my health; help me find loopholes; and help me get through the loopholes or at least not interfere.

I wanted her to take initiative, be creative, and apply her analytical skills to the system as much as to medicine. For example, I would have preferred that she tell me how to fit the inclusion and exclusion criteria. Or that she find out about the MCV test and alert me that there was a way for her to monitor whether I was taking AZT without putting it in my record.

These are high-level expectations. Quite advanced. You communicate them just like the rest, however — the other parts of the job description. Communicating these and other expectations requires persistence and follow-through on your part. It is not a one-shot deal with doctors any more than with other important people in your life.

Essentially, this means:
1) Remember that you, not the doctor, are the decision maker.
2) Keep your doctor's job description in mind.
3) Bring an agenda to appointments.
4) Never forget that your doctor has not been trained to deal with patients who follow numbers 1, 2, or 3 above!
5) Keep training your doctor. Training is an ongoing process.

And this brings us to our next subject ... MONITORING PERFORMANCE.

Before we go on, however, I've attached a sample agenda. After reading it, try drafting a sample agenda for communicating *your* expectations.

SAMPLE AGENDA
Date

1) CHAT WITH HIM, e.g., *"My ... how pretty you look today!"*

2) MOTIVATE HIM, e.g., *"Thanks for getting that letter to disability so quickly. I get so stressed out with all that complicated paperwork."*

3) MONITOR HIM. Review last month's unanswered questions, e.g., *"What did Doc Rayon say about mixing AZT, ddI, and marijuana as an effective treatment?"*

"Did you get the reference materials on the efficacy of interferon from the computer database?"

4) COMMUNICATE EXPECTATIONS CLEARLY, e.g., *"I must have misunderstood you. I thought you said interferon did not have serious side effects, other than flu-like symptoms. But I read in* Project Inform *that interferon causes impotence in 78 percent of patients. Can we talk about this?"*

5) MAKE YOUR NEEDS CLEAR, e.g., *"I need a Valium prescription."*

DOCTOR'S ACTION ITEMS
    1) Last month's unanswered questions
    2) This month's unanswered questions
    3) New requests

MONITORING PERFORMANCE

As you have seen, people with HIV encounter all sorts of administrative complications. In my view, it was my doctor's job to resolve administrative screwups. Millie's perspective, on the other hand, was, "I'm a doctor, not a secretary!" Not surprisingly, our differing expectations led to some conflict that we had to work through.

It was the end of September, 1989, a few weeks after Millie submitted my ddI application. The ddI had not arrived. I called Millie from my office and found that she hadn't taken any action. I told her that this situation was unacceptable.

"Give me your doctor ID number and *I'll* call Bristol-Myers," I exclaimed, exasperated. *"Somebody* has to follow up on this." She relented and called the company. She didn't want to hand out her ID number.

The first shipment of ddI arrived in early October. Soon my health stabilized and it later began to improve.

At the end of the October, I was running out of ddI and had not received the next batch from Bristol-Myers. They liked to wait until the last moment and then use Federal Express.

I wanted Millie to [can you guess?] take initiative and follow up before my supply was gone. She really didn't like following up on logistics, especially that level of detail. As it happened, I subsequently cut back to a half dose, which allowed me gradually to build up a large stockpile of ddI. This buffer stock made me less vulnerable to the haphazard shipment practices of Bristol-Myers. I'd solved the logistical problem.

Millie's performance problem, on the other hand, was lack of initiative. I wanted her to prevent problems before they happened, or at least to fix problems as they arose. It's like a banquet coordinator who learns that twenty-five extra guests have arrived at the Sheraton for the annual Elks Dinner. The hotel manager expects him to order extra meals and get tables set.

Millie quickly realized that there were rudimentary administrative things to attend to. Apparently her other HIV patients told her about troubles with lost blood tests and the switchboard. She adjusted her expectations and came up with simple solutions like giving out her page number.

In other cases, like checking with Bristol-Myers on my ddI application, she balked. "Doctors don't do this!" she announced. Well, my health depended on her doing those things. Clearly this wasn't what Millie envisioned back in medical school. But it's what needed to be done.

In fact, Millie has become an outstanding medical coordinator. She got me ddI. She has the forms; she keeps track of administrative things on her computer tickler file; and she writes excellent letters, very professional and informative, as required. She's become a good administrator. Mind you, she had to be trained and motivated.

Just for my own pleasure, I've designed a little report card for Millie. Here it is:

MEDICAL COORDINATOR SCHOOL
REPORT CARD

PUPIL'S NAME: Millie
TEACHER: Bob
SCHOOL: Beth Israel Hospital, Boston, Mass.

GROWTH OF SKILLS AND KNOWLEDGE

	1989	1990	1991
Analytical Skills	D	C-	C+
Administrative Skills	B	B+	A-
Computer Skills	C+	B	A
Initiative	F	C-	B-
Cooperation	C-	B+	A-

Comments:

First Reporting Period (1989): *Millie has made a good start. With continued effort, her initiative and computer skills can improve. Millie excels in the art of procrastination.*

Second Reporting Period (1990): *Improvement! Millie and I are both cautiously optimistic. Millie almost lost her "C" in Initiative last month.*

Third Reporting Period (1991): *Good Work! Millie seems eager to please. Promoted to "Colleague!"*

MOTIVATING YOUR DOCTOR

When to act EMPOWERED and when to act h-e-l-p-l-e-s-s? That is the question. If you're going to motivate your doctor, you have to get this.

I've been rather slow on this point. I was almost forty before I figured out that if you yell at hospital staff they just get defensive. It's like managing your boss. When he's making you crazy, first you point out things he's doing well, *then* you discuss the problem areas.

With Millie, I was tearing my hair out for months. I wanted her to *care* about taking initiative, to *want* to do it. That was the issue: She wasn't *motivated* to take initiative.

This insight came to me via my therapist, Andre, who pointed out that doctors are people, too. To get motivated, doctors have to feel they're *helping* you. You must say, "Oh you've been so helpful in writing my disability letter" or in getting ddI. That encourages them to do more. It's called positive reinforcement.

Andre and I discussed this in numerous sessions. Well, I got it and got better at it. For example, I learned to approach the receptionists and lab techs by saying, "Oh, I don't know what to do. I'm so upset. Maybe you can help!" I was amazed; they wanted to help! Not always, of course.

You must use simple psychology. Listen to them. Ask what they think and why. When they do something right, say, "Ooh, ya did a good job!" When they do something bad, you have to be real firm. And remember, change takes time.

Of course, when I later told Andre, "Oh, you've been so helpful, Andre. This has really helped me work with Millie," he did give me a funny look.

You also have to know how to fire your doctor. Generally you just stop seeing him.

The funny part is that usually when you hire people, they expect you to fill the role of manager, although a lot of them resent it. But doctors think *they're* in control and *we're* the subordinates. They don't understand that we *hire* them and *pay* them. They are consultants, not bosses.

When you hire a plumber, he does what you decide to have done. When you hire a lawyer, she is supposed to do what you want. And when you hire a doctor, he should give you professional advice, like a consultant, but ultimately he should do what you want.

Doctors use a different logic, however. They're still in the fifties. They expect you to say, "Oh, Doctor, help me, help me! I know nothing! Tell me what to do!" We're the fifties housewives and they're the husbands. They work in the Real World, and our job is to be cute and cooperative.

Well, it's not the fifties any more. We've been liberated and empowered. Of course, many doctors think patients have become too empowered.

Doctors don't like being supervised. They don't like anyone monitoring their behavior. Who does? Doctors don't like being held accountable. Who ever heard of holding a doctor accountable? When is the last time the AMA censured a doctor? Lawyers will tell you that fear of malpractice suits — and all the procedures designed to minimize them — keeps doctors accountable. That's baloney. Malpractice suits happen because doctors are not managed.

What if your accountant didn't get your forms into the IRS on time? I bet you'd say something to him. When the doctor doesn't get a piece of information he is supposed to get, why shouldn't you demand it? At least ask for it again. And keep track of what was supposed to be done.

The erroneous assumption of people who don't supervise their doctors is that doctors remember your questions and follow up on their own. But they don't! They forget. And no wonder — with five hundred or a thousand patients, they're busy and distractible.

You want them to make the best possible use of the time they do set aside for you. Don't assume they'll make time to reflect and plan. Set priorities with them and then follow up. You're the one with the time — or at least the one who has to find the time. Invest some of that time in managing your doctor, so that he uses *his* time and skills to better meet your needs.

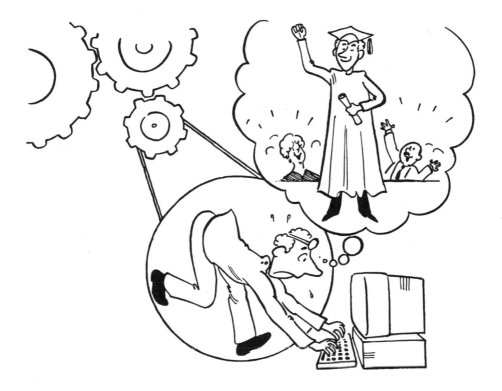

MORAL: **Hire a doctor with good administrative skills.**
Those skills are the keys to the system.

6

Obtaining Experimental Drugs

When established drugs and therapies are not working for you, it's time to consider other options: experimental drugs.

People use phrases like *"applying* for experimental drugs." This makes the process sound like applying for college. You fill out an application and they let you in or they don't. Simple.

Well, it's not simple at all. Obtaining experimental drugs is more like buying a house:

1) There are many parties involved, each with distinct and differing objectives.

2) Your exact objective — to buy the house or to obtain the drug — is held by no one else, not even people who work with or for you.

3) There is an exchange. You must give something in order to receive.

4) To negotiate successfully, *you must understand the differing objectives of each player in the game.*

Here are some questions you may be thinking about:
- When should I consider experimental drugs?
- How do I find out about them?
- How do I choose one?
- Who gets chosen for studies? Who gets excluded?
- How do I learn about efficacy, dosage, and side effects?
- What tests will I be required to take?
- How long will I have to remain on the study? Can I stop?
- If the study is terminated, can I continue receiving the drug?

- What is the probability that I will get the real drug? A placebo?
- Will I be able to tell if I'm getting the placebo? How?
- Will I be given a dose that's too high? Can I control the dosage?
- Can I get experimental drugs without joining a study?

Before I introduce you to the Experimental Drug Game, let me repeat: Your objective is to stay alive and healthy for as long as possible. *No one in the HIV system but YOU has your health and longevity as a primary objective.*

STEP ONE: REALIZING YOU NEED A BIGGER HOUSE (Your treatment's not working)

Staying alive with HIV means shopping for appropriate drugs and therapies. It's like trying to furnish your house at a mall where the sales staff (doctors, in this case) are poorly trained and managed.

- They don't know what's available in other sections of the mall;
- They don't focus on your needs; and
- They all give you the hard sell for their particular product (radiation, chemo, drugs, and so on).

Sometimes, however, your problem can't be solved by redecorating. The neighborhood has gone to hell. You need a different house.

That was my situation in May 1989, when I had clearly stopped responding to AZT.

I started taking AZT in 1987. When I did, my health stabilized. I also began reading about ddI, which had just been mentioned in the press. It looked promising: less toxic and basically a better version of AZT. (Whenever I start a new treatment, I try to look ahead to the next, because most treatments are only effective for so long. There's a point after which you don't respond any more. This is true for AZT and it may be true for ddI, too.)

Anyway, AZT was no longer working. I was losing weight and my KS started running amok, first on my legs, then everywhere: arms, chest, lungs, internal organs. The oncologists and Infectious Disease docs put me on interferon in May. That made me really sick — and didn't seem to have any effect on my lesions — so I stopped after four weeks. Next they urged me to try other kinds of chemotherapy.

My house was on fire and my homeowner's policy had lapsed! I decided to pursue radiation, in the short run, to put out the fire. I had to get my legs under control. After all, radiation had worked before.

The Radiation Therapy receptionist said the first available appointment was in two months. Yes, she understood my leg was falling off. The first opening was in August. At my next oncology appointment, I asked Bubbles to call Radiation Therapy and make them understand the urgency of my situation. He consented so halfheartedly that I didn't believe he would follow through.

"Look," I said, "I'll go over there right now. Wait five minutes and *call them.*" Then I ran over to Radiation Therapy, in the next building, right to the receptionist who had told me, "You'll just have to wait."

I pulled up my pant leg, revealing masses of large lesions, and said in a loud voice, "Look at this!" The receptionist leaned over to look down, eyebrows raised, and said into the phone, "Uh-huh, here he is right now!" An incredulous doctor was observing this scene. He motioned to me and said, "I'll see you in ten minutes." That's how I got started on radiation therapy. We radiated my legs daily (Monday through Friday) for three weeks. By early July, they looked like I'd been walking on the sun.

In the meantime, I investigated ddI more closely. I didn't really have a plan of action, but my objective was clear: Get ddI or find a better drug. I took it step by step, gathering information and investigating options, loopholes, and so forth. Ultimately I found the loophole I mentioned in chapter 5: Bristol-Myers would give ddI on a "compassionate-use" basis to PWAs experiencing rapid weight loss. I knew to focus on this angle with my doctor. But that's getting ahead of the story.

I needed information on the efficacy and availability of ddI. Where would you turn if you didn't have confidence in the information you were getting from the doctors? Your local AIDS service organization (ASO), of course. Since I was on staff at my local organization, you would think I would be reasonably well connected. Well, I was.

I thought of my advocate, Taffy, who was burned out and

would be leaving AIDS Action in a couple months. Back in 1986, you'll remember, I approached Taffy for information on the efficacy of chemotherapy. He told me about brown rice and granola! In the intervening three years, Taffy had learned a bit about treatments, so I thought I might try him again. One morning I bumped into him on my way into the office and said, "Taffy, I may need to get ddI. How do I do make the switch?"

"From what I know," he yawned, "the studies are closed." He really didn't care to know about anything medical. Like other client advocates, he had a fear of medical things that was absolutely eye-popping.

Well, the Phase One studies had indeed closed to further enrollment in the summer of 1989. But the Phase Two studies were gearing up. Some had started — but not all. Taffy was giving me misinformation, which was not unusual.

What appalled me was his lack of initiative. He didn't say, "Oh, I'll see what I can do. Let me look into it." Anyway, I knew not to deal with Taffy any more.

Shortly thereafter, I was chatting with Taffy's boss, Daddy Earl. Earl was director of client services and reported to me. He kept his office dark, lit only by a desk lamp. I thought it was soothing and — given some of his excitable staff — appropriate.

"Earl," I began, "I want to ask you to think about something. But I want you to listen to me as a person with AIDS, not as your boss."

"Sure, Bob." He clasped his hands and waited.

"Don't you think, at this point in the epidemic, we should be able to give people with AIDS information about experimental drugs that might keep them alive?" I told him about my experience with Taffy.

He chuckled. "You know Taffy. But he tries. And most of his clients seem to like him. He really cares."

"But what about the medical information?"

"I'm thinking of having a volunteer give us some medical updates. But the advocates are so busy. Besides, they don't have medical training and this stuff produces a lot of anxiety."

I didn't like the direction this was taking. "I don't think their fear should be the issue here, Earl!"

At this point, Earl switched tack.

"I know, I know. But there's been a big wave of illness recently and I don't want to add to the stress. You must be angry about being sick again, Bob, too."

"Yes I am angry, but that's not what this is about. Don't talk about my being an angry PWA. That's avoiding the issue."

He looked surprised. "Okay. I'll look into it. In the meantime, I have something for you. It's a new benefit we're offering clients." He winked and gave me a free access code to a phone sex line.

Somewhat boggled, I thanked him and left. When I asked for medical information, I got misinformation — and an offer of free phone sex. When I tried to hold the system accountable, I was manipulated. It was time to pursue other avenues.

STEP TWO: SHOPPING FOR THE NEW HOUSE, or Gathering Information

You, the patient, have more time and more motivation to research experimental drugs than your doctor does. You also have critical information that she lacks. You know your body better — or should. In particular, you know in detail how you responded to previous drugs.

These resources are critical, but they are not enough. It also takes system-sense to gather information on experimental drugs. By definition, the drugs are new, so information is fragmented and harder to find. Moreover, not everyone wants to share the information you need.

The reason for this — and some solutions — are contained in my theory of differing objectives.

I've already made the analogy that getting an experimental drug is like buying a house. Each player has distinct objectives. These objectives are rarely stated up front.

When you buy a house, you must deal with a bank. By lending money, the bank makes a profit and you gain access to your new house. In order to lend money, bank management has certain roles and responsibilities, including stringent regulations it must follow. Hospitals and other medical facilities are the medical equivalent of banks. They control access to experimental drug protocols, which are also called clinical trials.

Inside the hospital is the gatekeeper to the protocol, Maggie, in my case. This manager is analogous to the loan officer at the bank. Getting you the loan is not her primary objective. In her view, it would be nice if you obtained your loan, but her salary and her performance review won't be hurt if you are rejected. Her priority is screening out the bad risks!

The primary care physician is like your lawyer. The lawyer is the only one working for you — sort of. She wants to help you purchase your house. And the job of my primary care physician, Millie, is to help me get experimental drugs. While the lawyer doesn't want to break rules, she's not as stringent as the loan officer, who in turn is not as stringent as bank management. Similarly, Millie was not as stringent as Maggie, who was in turn not as stringent as the hospital.

The hospital and the doctors are afraid they'll get sued for malpractice. Their objective is to avoid suit and stay in business. To this end, hospitals have created legal departments, review committees, procedures, and guidelines. Sometimes the guidelines are outrageous. For example, Beth Israel's guidelines forbid doctors from discussing your lover's medical care with you, even if he's dying, unless you've met certain requirements, like a living will. Clearly, in an emergency, those guidelines can conflict with your objective, which is caring for the welfare of your lover.

Now we come to the real estate agents, who make money on the transactions. Sleazy operators, whose primary objective is to make as many transactions happen as possible. Who in the medical system parallels the real estate agents?

The drug companies!

They care about making money. They are not accountable for, and don't care about, your individual health or welfare. Nor do they care about people with HIV on the whole. At each stage of the game, whether it's demonstrating efficacy or minimizing toxicity, drug companies do what they can to get their drugs licensed and accelerate profits.

Take the final approval of Bristol-Myers's ddI, for example. The competing drug, AZT, is manufactured by Burroughs Wellcome. Burroughs Wellcome knew its AZT sales and profits would drop as soon as ddI was approved by the FDA. Do you suppose that Burroughs Wellcome might have had an interest in slowing down the ddI approval process? Just like one real estate agent trying to subvert another agent who is competing for a customer?

These, then, are some of the principle players in the Experimental Drug Game: the hospital (test site), the protocol coordinator, your primary care physician, and the drug manufacturer.

Through my reading — *Project Inform, GMHC Treatment News,* and so forth — I knew that various hospitals around the country would be participating in the Phase Two trials of ddI — and that Boston's Beth Israel was one of them. That's why I got a primary care physician — to help me coordinate the application process.

In other words, I decided to go through proper channels. As it turned out, the first doctor I got was Dr. Cornfield — a dud. It would be a month or two before I finally got Millie. In the meantime, I had to do things on my own. Keep in mind, I was getting sicker all the time.

I began by lining up appointments with Infectious Disease docs at Beth Israel — Doc Rayon, Clark Kent, and Maggie: the whole chain of command. These are some of the most renowned Infectious Disease people in New England. The ones who give the speeches.

Doc Rayon was the first one. How shall I describe her? Rigid, emotionless, stone-faced. Rayon projected an attitude of "Why bother, you're gonna die." She told me, very simply, "It's not likely that ddI will help you, and you're not qualified." Period. Zum Ende. That was that.

Rayon's opinion, later echoed by Maggie, was that I should seek more aggressive chemotherapy.

To both of them I said, "But I've seen over and over, at this stage of the disease, people who do chemotherapy die within a few months!" Nonetheless, they both insisted that chemo was the only option.

Now, when a doctor insists you do something — that it's your only option — what would you assume? That it's probably going to help you, right? Well, I knew the probability was *enormous* that chemo would kill me and very *slim* that it would help. And I knew that Maggie knew it, too, but was pretending otherwise!

This issue was too important to leave unspoken. I asked Maggie to tell me the probability that I would respond to chemotherapy.

"I don't have that number offhand."

"Hmm," I responded, "you *do* know that the probability of chemotherapy working the first time is 50 to 60 percent, right?"

"Yes," she said.

"And the second time, it's less, isn't it?"

"Yes."

"And it goes down each time thereafter, right?"

She nodded.

"Well, this will be my sixth bout of chemo. So would you guess the probability of my responding positively would be around 10 percent?"

"Maybe," she admitted grudgingly.

"Well, what do you think the probability would be that I'll respond to ddI?"

"I have absolutely no way to estimate that."

"Could it be greater than 10 percent?"

"I just can't respond to that!" she said flatly.

"Well," I replied, "I bet it *is* greater than 10 percent and I want to take that risk."

Maggie and Rayon were recommending I follow the Approved Procedure at that time: When AZT stops working, go to Chemo. Do not pass Go. But I knew the approved procedure was not in my best interest. Chemo would have killed me. It has killed several friends since then.

Let me tell you the whole story of my meeting with Maggie. It will show you how drastically the differing objectives of various doctors can impede your search for effective treatment. First, however, let me share a little guide I made to clarify the objectives of the players in the Experimental Treatment Game.

EXPERIMENTAL DRUG SHOPPER'S GUIDE

BUYING A NEW HOUSE	OBTAINING AN EXPERIMEN- TAL DRUG	OBJECTIVE(S):
REALTOR	DRUG COMPANY	Make as much money possible
YOUR LAWYER	YOUR DOCTOR	1) Don't lose license 2) Don't get sued 3) Look out for your welfare
THE BANK	THE HOSPITAL	1) Stay in business 2) Follow regulations and procedures, with little flexibility
APPRAISOR	BLOOD LAB	Follow the procedures, no matter how stupid
BANK REGULATORS	THE FDA	1) Document that they won't repeat the previous disaster 2) Maintain political power
CONSUMER PROTECTION AGENCY	YOUR LOCAL AIDS SERVICE ORGANIZATION	1) Head off stupid legislation 2) Don't piss off funding sources 3) Look out for welfare of individual clients

Your objective as a patient is to stay alive for as long as possible and to stay as healthy as possible. Can you see how the objectives of other players might lead to conflict?

Maggie was an Infectious Disease doctor who understood HIV and followed ddI. I wanted her opinion — and support, if possible. Maggie knew which populations were more likely to respond to ddI. She knew about efficacy, dosage, and so forth — the medical stuff. She also knew the system, because she was working with Bristol-Myers on the ddI Phase Two study. She controlled entrance to the ddI protocols. She was a gate-keeper — the loan officer, as it were. I later came to realize that this meant her objective was to limit access to the protocol.

Getting an appointment with Maggie was virtually impossible. Running the ddI study was fast becoming a full-time job. Word was out that ddI looked good, so there were lots of eager applicants. Maggie was very popular.

I had no primary care physician to refer me to Maggie or advocate for me, so I plotted with Larry Killian. If I couldn't obtain an appointment with Maggie concerning ddI, maybe Larry could get one, on more-normal Infectious Disease business. For over a year, he had been plagued by large itchy bumps on his arms and legs. Two biopsies had revealed nothing. Now the warmer weather seemed to be aggravating the bumps. Larry complained strenuously to his primary care physician — and was able to get a July appointment to see Maggie.

We choreographed the appointment beforehand. First, Larry would focus on the bumps. What were they and why wouldn't they go away? The idea was for me to go along — we told Maggie I'd be coming — "and by the way, Maggie, what about ddI?"

Picture Maggie: five-feet-four, curly hair, intelligent, articulate, and an ego as big as a house. A control queen. Reminded me of myself, actually.

Larry introduced us before reviewing the history of his bumps. Maggie had no idea what they were. She wanted to cut them out and biopsy them for the third time and find nothing. You know how they do that. We talked about invasive procedures in chapter 3.

Larry decided to forego the biopsy and continue with his ointments. Then he said, "Bob is thinking of doing ddI. And I may be also."

"I see," she responded. "Well, the Phase One results don't look that good: It causes pancreatitis and neuropathy. Very serious stuff, you know."

Pancreatitis is an inflammation of the pancreas. Neuropathy is nerve damage in your hands and feet.

"But the intent of the Phase One studies," I observed, "is to find those toxicities. They keep giving you enough ddI until they find them, right?"

"Yes, we've found the toxicities and they're there!"

"Isn't it possible they won't occur at lower doses?"

"I can't risk that," she said.

That stopped me for a moment. *She's giving me an instant no,* I thought, *but based on what? What kind of risk are we talking about? And how big is the risk? Compared to what?*

"The dosages being given to people on Phase Two are a fraction of the Phase One doses," I continued. "What if I took even less than the Phase Two dose, given what we know about AZT?"

Burroughs Wellcome had tested AZT at a very high dose in the Phase Two trials: 1200 mg. I reduced my AZT dosage to 600 mg early on and later to 300 mg — long before Burroughs Wellcome told people to do so. My theory was that the Phase Two dosage was similarly high for ddI. I was asking Maggie if the same course of events might occur with ddI.

"But that's not how the studies work," protested Maggie.

Aha! I thought. *She's not talking about risks to* me. *She's thinking of risks to* her *as manager of the study.*

"I understand how the studies work," I rejoined. "But I'm trying to live. I'm trying to treat my disease as a chronic condition and *live.*"

Maggie was hung up on the scientific integrity of the study, as she should have been. It was her job. But here's the rub: Her job was also to keep out patients who were at risk for serious side effects, *even if they might well benefit from ddI.*

Maggie and Bristol-Myers wanted the patients ddI was most likely to help — and least likely to harm. The objective in Phase Two clinical trials is to determine optimum dosage — the dosage at which the most people show positive results. The drug companies don't want toxic reactions when they're trying to get FDA approval for a new drug. If you've had liver problems, for example, you're more likely to have a toxic reaction, even at a lower dose, so they want to keep you out of the Phase Two study.

None of those things had to do with my health. We had differing objectives.

We tussled another twenty minutes. Finally I just said, "Maggie, look at me. My legs look like French fries. And that's a success. I can't radiate the rest of me like this. I'm dying. I'm terminal at this point. Would you say I have three to six months left?"

"That could be," she admitted.

"So why not try it?! Even if there's only a 25 percent chance of my getting better, as opposed to the certainty of my dying, why not try it?"

She leaned forward and said earnestly, "I cannot risk giving you three more months of a little bit healthier life, possibly, against the potentially serious and very painful side effects. The neuropathy, pancreatitis, and so forth."

I bridled. "What do you mean, *you* can't risk it. How dare you make that decision! It's not your risk!"

At this point, Maggie drew herself up and stated, "I'm the doctor. This is my *job!*"

"No!" I said emphatically. "You may be the doctor, but this is *not* your decision. You're *consulting* to me: giving me advice and information. The bottom line is, it's *my* decision."

I was incensed. I paused, searching for another way to make contact. I wanted Maggie to focus on my health — not the protocol.

After a moment, I continued, "Maggie, let me throw you something else. Let's assume availability is not an issue. Assume we're outside of this protocol and Phase Two business; you have no responsibilities for this study. And assume I'm your brother. Would you recommend I try ddI?"

"I can't answer that question!" she said. "It's too hypothetical."

When dealing with drugs and doctors, I advise friends with HIV to set aside the issues of accessibility and availability. Doctors and patients get overwhelmed with logistics of the system and lose sight of the key issue. First decide if you want to take the drug, *then* deal with how to get it. Separate the issues and focus on the medical question first. I was asking Maggie to do just that. She couldn't. Or wouldn't.

"You realize that we have some differing objectives here," I said.

"And you have to understand," she replied coolly, "that I'm responsible for the integrity of this process here."

"But I'm talking about getting ddI via compassionate use now!"

I knew, of course, that data is also collected on patients receiving experimental drugs under compassionate use. I was not an attractive candidate. Maggie knew I was considering chemo and therefore more likely to have complications. If I took ddI and had medical complications — whether related to ddI or not — the FDA and Bristol-Myers would ask more questions down the road. She wanted to minimize those hassles.

I was angry. I had worked hard to explain my logic to her and she was offended. I had challenged her. My logic made sense and she wouldn't even respond. As we left, Larry grunted thoughtfully.

"Now I understand what you've been saying about differing objectives," he mused. "You really have to take matters into your own hands."

Many people think that doctors are there exclusively to cure you. They're not. Although they truly want to help you, their first obligation — to the system and to their other patients — is to respect the rules and stay in business. Doctors are there to do a job. Maggie's job was to manage entry to the protocol. Period. That objective outweighed everything else, including my health. She'd done everything she could to discourage me — and told me nothing about the system.

A few days later, David Aronstein at AIDS Action told me he'd spotted an announcement about an upcoming seminar for primary care physicians at Beth Israel on, of all things, recruiting appropriate subjects for clinical trials. The presenter was to be ... Maggie!

David went with me on a late July evening. We noted a couple of other PWAs in the audience. As Maggie discussed inclusion and exclusion criteria, a bell went off and I realized this was something I needed to study carefully. The heart of her talk was about how to keep people out.

Maggie looked my way a couple times, expecting trouble. She didn't like my being there. But I knew I had a right to attend: FDA regulations made the meeting public. And I'm smart enough not to make a scene with all the doctors together in one room. I sat there quietly taking notes and I learned some interesting stuff.

For example, I had only a two-thirds chance of receiving ddI if I were accepted into the protocol. That was bad news. One-third of the subjects would receive AZT, which I already knew did me no good. The good news? Maggie described a blood test called MCV that can indicate the presence of AZT in the bloodstream. Knowing this, I could take an MCV test and drop out of the protocol if I discovered I was getting AZT.

After the seminar, David and I discussed what we'd learned. The system was complicated — it seemed to have loopholes, like the MCV test — but loopholes take time to exploit. The protocol would not start until the autumn. Assuming I were accepted, I had only a 67 percent probability of getting ddI. It would take another month to determine if they'd actually slipped me AZT. Then I'd have to set about getting ddI all over. I wanted a 100 percent probability of getting ddI — and soon.

"Compassionate use" was the route to pursue and I knew too little about it. I wanted to know more about "shopping for a bigger house," namely, who gets ddI on "compassionate use," how, and why? I contacted a friend at the state Department of Public Health. We had met two years earlier, when he volunteered with me on the Information Systems needs assessment for AIDS Action. He sent me the inclusion and exclusion criteria, which I studied.

Here's what I learned.

If you didn't qualify for the formal study, you could request ddI on a compassionate-use basis, providing you met certain conditions:

1) You couldn't tolerate AZT. It was making you sick, i.e., anemic, nauseated, etc.; or

2) You had stopped responding to AZT.

Unfortunately, as I recounted earlier, the official list of symptoms which constituted "no longer responding to AZT" did not include raging KS. The list was new and incomplete.

I probably would not get ddI under the compassionate-use program unless I somehow lied. I had started losing weight, so the weight loss angle looked like a possibility. As I thought over my strategy, I realized Maggie could have hinted about the weight loss inclusion criterion, since she knew the protocol in detail. She had done nothing helpful. She totally lacked human qualities.

One doctor tried to be helpful: Clark Kent, whom I talked to after Rayon and before Maggie. Clark was unassuming, five-feet-nine, and dark-haired. He reminded me of Superman's alter ego, hence the nickname. I admired his big thighs and theorized that there might be something worth seeing under those clothes.

Clark was the only doctor who even hinted that ddI might be a good idea. When I said, "Let's assume that availability is not a problem; let's just focus on the medical issue," Clark was the only one willing to engage with me.

I said, "Clark, you know that I can get ddI under the table if I have to. Do you think it might be worth a shot? If I were your brother, what would you tell me?"

"I would tell you to do it," he replied.

Clark was not a typical Infectious Disease doc. He identified with his patients and was willing to view them as peers. What were Clark's objectives? I'm not sure. Clearly, he was not wedded to the hospital system. He was very sympathetic.

As you can see, differing objectives affect how people think and talk, how much they reveal, and what they choose to conceal. Watch for differing objectives, especially when they aren't stated up front. Here are a few phrases which should make bells go off in your head.

PHRASES TO LOOK OUT FOR ... AND POSSIBLE RESPONSES

Don't you trust me?	I don't trust my mother, may she rest in peace!
We've done all we can do	You've done all you *want* to do.
This is the only option	But I read in the newspaper about this other option...
That information is not available	How do we get it?

That's not my job	Whose job is it?
You don't qualify	Make me qualify! What do I have to do?
Don't worry about the side effects	May I please speak to a nurse?
That's the procedure	Fuck the procedure!

STEP THREE: APPLYING FOR A MORTGAGE, or Submitting the Right Paperwork

When you ask the bank for a mortgage, your debt-to-income ratio must be less than 28 percent. In other words, if you make $25,000 a year, your annual debt payments may not exceed $7,000 (7000/25,000 = 28%). The loan officer doesn't want to hear or see a number higher than that. If she does, you're not qualified. Furthermore, you must be able to make the down payment out of your own savings; none of it can be borrowed.

Now, we all know people who've borrowed money for their down payment, whether from Mummy and Daddy or from VISA. And they don't record that loan on their mortgage application, nor do they mention it to their lawyers. Why? Because they keep in mind how their objectives, as the home buyers, differ from those of the loan officer.

Similarly, the application process for experimental drugs involves complicated paperwork and many players. Blood tests, medical history, drug history, and so forth. The company wants to know all sorts of things. And *you* want to qualify. What will get you into the study and what will keep you out?

The inclusion and exclusion criteria provide the answers.

Inclusion criteria are characteristics the drug company wants to see in the guinea pigs. They'll want a diagnosis of AIDS, a certain level of T4 cells, and so on.

Exclusion criteria are the opposite: They are the red flags that tell the company you're undesirable. For example, patients receiving chemo are commonly excluded from protocols. Why? Because the chemo damages your immune system temporarily, making you prone to infections. The drug company doesn't want its guinea pigs getting sick due to chemo and having it blamed on their new drug. Knowing that, you *defer* your chemotherapy until after you've applied for the study. Otherwise, you close off your option. It's like not buying the new car until you've bought the house.

Your primary care physician is like your lawyer. She is the most closely tied to you; she wants you to be healthy. But she can't violate the law. And she has certain career objectives. If she is a resident (they're students, really) she wants to show that she can handle cases by herself. Frankly though, residents can't do it all by themselves — not when it comes to a complex disease like AIDS. They're not unlike junior employees in a computer department who say, "I'm gonna do it myself. I know how to do it." But they don't.

When *I* was a junior computer programmer for a large insurance company, for example, I was assigned to design a daily check-balancing system. I did it all by myself. Unfortunately, the program I wrote took twenty-six hours to run.

If you keep in mind how loosely doctors are supervised, you'll realize that it's up to you to prod the resident to seek out a specialist and get a higher level opinion. Differing objectives...

Anyway, back to inclusion and exclusion criteria. I had to mull over these criteria. It's harder for me, since I'm not a doctor. In particular, it took time to study the assumptions behind the ddI protocol. Doctors already know the assumptions. Unfortunately, they're not trained to discuss them with you. They take them for granted.

Because I had prepared in this way, I was ready later, when my new doctor, Millie, and I opened the plastic on *her* packet of materials.

"Look here, Millie," I said, "it says you qualify if you're not responding to AZT. And look! One sign of not responding is rapid weight loss. Eight pounds in a month! Do you think that could happen to me? What would happen if I lost eight pounds in a month?"

Millie was at a bit of a loss. She was unfamiliar with these application procedures and how the criteria might apply to me. She was overwhelmed with paperwork and logistics, as we all were. Moreover, she expected I was going to die anyway. She had a thousand patients and this seemed like a waste of time. Three years later, she's more experienced and she knows it's not a waste of time.

Since I already knew I was going for the weight loss angle, I had set the stage accordingly. Before my appointment, I'd had Nurse Doozie weigh me and I was as heavy as could be. I'd eaten a lobster dinner the night before, was wearing a heavy coat even though it was a warm September day, and held onto my briefcase while standing on the scale.

That part — the briefcase — was really special! Doozie just put me on the scale as if she couldn't care less about her job. She didn't like what she was doing. She didn't like the doctors. They made more money than her. She didn't care for fags. And dealing with me was just one more nuisance.

No, not pleasant. Not a happy person. Not a motivated person.

So you take advantage of that. If you know they're not going to do their job properly, that can be an opportunity! I didn't have to hide weights in my pants. I could just wear my coat and hold my briefcase. So everybody wins! A win-win situation! America!

Anyway, I told Millie, "Look, I've been losing weight recently — and rather fast. Let's see what happens." As I left, I had the receptionist schedule an appointment for one week later, rather than one month. Then I went on a crash diet.

The following week, famished, I had Doozie weigh me again. I actually measured only seven pounds lighter, even though I was wearing practically nothing. In her office a few minutes later, Millie studied Doozie's handwriting and mentally calculated my weight loss. I glared at her and said through clenched teeth, "Make it eight pounds!" Reluctantly, she subtracted the extra pound. We were under way!

We began assembling my application. As I described earlier, this meant documenting previous treatments and taking dozens of blood tests. And dealing with the elves down in the blood lab.

The hospital lab can be compared to the real estate appraiser. The appraiser follows established procedures to assign a value to your property. His objective is to conform to procedures, even if it means overlooking unique aspects of your property. You, on the other hand, want the appraised value to be as high as possible. The blood bank wants to assess your blood. Their objective is to follow the procedures, no matter how stupid. My objective as patient is to have my blood look as good as possible so I can get the drug. I want it to conform to the experimental requirements.

The purpose of the compassionate-use program was to help people who would die without ddI, but might live if they got it. That described *me*. My body had responded to another antiviral, AZT, which checked my lesions for a long time. I had no significant side effects — my bone marrow had been superb. I reasoned that it wasn't critical that I meet the criteria on *each* blood test; I thought it would be okay if I were a little out of range on a couple. What was more important was the likelihood I would respond to antivirals, hence ddI. *I needed the ddI and would probably benefit from it.*

That was the spirit behind the compassionate-use program, but the system did not operate according to my logic. The rules weren't meant to hurt people, but sometimes they did.

STEP FOUR: CLOSING THE DEAL, or Managing Details

When closing on your house, all sorts of documents have to come together at the same time: title search, mortgage, inspections, insurance, etc. Any one of a number of faceless clerks can lose paperwork and hold up the deal. At which point *you* don't have a place to live, while they just go on about business as usual.

The experienced home buyer knows that his job is to make sure this doesn't happen.

Similarly, the clerks at the hospital frequently lose blood tests and other paperwork. And the drug company staff are no better.

It's your job to track that. None of these people are actually held accountable for follow-through. The primary care physician's *real job* is to do some of it, but not all of it.

Over time, treating HIV is getting more and more complicated. More drugs, more protocols, more procedures, more information. The medical community, after all, is getting more sophisticated. And patients with HIV are going to have to get more sophisticated in managing the process. The drug companies, for example, are closing the loopholes. In trials of upcoming drugs they probably won't allow patients with HIV into their seminars. So we'll have to find other ways to get the information. And we will.

STEP FIVE: SETTLING INTO THE NEW HOUSE, or Adjusting to the New Drug

Once you get the experimental drug, you have to settle in, just like with a new house. Things never work quite the way you expect.

In a new home, you have to figure out the appliances and how to regulate the heat. You need to get homeowners insurance; handle the telephone installation; and attend to change-of-address screwups.

Likewise, with a new drug, you'll need to:
- assure a regular supply;
- tinker with the dosage and the timing of the dosage; and
- manage the side effects.

Don't think for a minute that the system either wants to, or can, do this for you. It's your job.

My first month on ddI, I took the full dose, as recommended, to get a good hit into my system. As warned, I developed diarrhea. I also developed heartburn. When I cut back to a half dose in November, the diarrhea diminished, but it still bothered me.

Of course, Millie wanted me to continue taking the full dose. She told me, "Bristol-Myers says take two packs a day. How can you mess with the dosage? I'm the doctor and I say take the two packs a day. Why won't you listen to me?"

This was October 1989. Stuff like the dosage patterns in Phase One and Phase Two — all that was new information to her.

I explained that the drug companies use a higher dose because they can show efficacy faster, with more patients. I also explained that I wanted to treat my disease chronically rather than terminally. I wanted to take the minimum effective dose — which no one yet knew — so that I would still be around in a couple years when the *next* drug came out! I wanted to minimize harmful — and possibly life-shortening — side effects.

I explained my logic and asked her to explain hers. Her

logic was, "This is what the FDA tells us to do. This is the *pro-cee-dure.*"

"That procedure makes sense within the framework of the FDA's drug approval process," I responded. "But it doesn't make sense in the context of *my* continuing-to-stay-alive process." Again, differing objectives!

Clearly we disagreed. But Millie knew better than to really argue with me. This was part of her training as an AIDS primary care physician, as I've recounted elsewhere. Today she understands that stuff.

For my diarrhea, Millie had been giving me Kaopectate. And Maalox for the heartburn. One day a light went off in her head. Maalox, which is widely used for heartburn, is a diuretic. It makes diarrhea worse! She had me stop taking the Kaopectate altogether and gave me Amphogel, an antacid which constipates. The heartburn stayed under control and the diarrhea diminished further.

Finally, I figured out that if you take ddI with lukewarm water, rather than cold water, as recommended, it mixes more easily and tastes less vile. I find a martini glass particularly effective.

Overall, the most important thing I did to manage the side effects was to cut back to half a dose. The point is, you deal with these things step by step, using common sense and trial-and-error. It's not unlike moving into a new house.

STEP SIX: TWO YEARS LATER, EVERYONE WANTS TO MOVE INTO THE NEIGHBORHOOD

When I started the ddI, in October 1989, my T4 count was 160. Six weeks later it was 260. My T4s climbed steadily to over 400 and they've been bouncing between 300 and 400 ever since. By Thanksgiving my lesions had stopped spreading, and by Christmas I was starting to feel better. After New Year's, my lesions began shrinking. They've continued to do so ever since.

In retrospect, it sounds like a rosy story. In fact, it was a close call that scared the daylights out of me. In July Maggie told me I had six months to live. When Millie received the first shipment of ddI, I figured I had three months left. I called Millie from the South Shore of Massachusetts, where I was attending my friend Bobby's memorial service on a Friday afternoon. I was so nervous about delaying until Monday that I left the service, drove into the city, and got the ddI.

For the next six weeks, my health was up and down. I was at home in bed more than I was at AIDS Action. The recruitment of a full-time deputy director was behind schedule. I told the board of directors they must hire my replacement by January 1. They did.

Although my health improved steadily after Christmas, I was quite sobered. As always, I wanted to be independent (read: *In control*). I saw that living in the country might restrict my independence, so I began looking for a place in Boston. I wanted to make life easier if and when I got sick. I wanted easy access to the hospital, to my friends, especially if they had to take care of me, and to shops and restaurants. I thought Mario would like being closer to his friends, too.

I had mixed feelings about moving. Mario and I loved our house in the woods. I would miss the stillness — and the deck. I also feared I was somehow giving up — accommodating myself to HIV — and didn't look forward to the hassle of moving. But Andre told me if I could handle running the nation's third-largest AIDS organization, I could handle moving back to the city.

Over the winter, my health improved steadily. I continued volunteering as a newly appointed member of the board of directors. Larry and I talked about starting a business together. We didn't know what we'd do, but we wanted it to be fun.

In midwinter I found a condo a couple miles from downtown. It fit the bill. The trolley stopped in front of the house. If I got too sick to drive, the hospital was just a short ride. The supermarket was a block away. I think of it as my walk-in refrigerator.

Mario and I moved in late April. I told myself, *I wish I were moving here to live for the next twenty years.* There was even room for an office, which I began sprucing up for my next career. Being in the city suited both Mario and me. Soon I took up bicycling again. The next summer, I took up rollerblading! A student doctor at Beth Israel saw my bruises from some early spills and thought they were lesions. I don't *have* any lesions that pronounced today.

Clark Kent examined me after eight months and said I'd

had the best response to ddI he'd seen. I believe that's because I started treatment with more T-cells than most people who get experimental AIDS drugs. Although I was sick, I had more of an immune system to work with. It may not work that way for everyone, but it's a good reason to push to start treatments early.

Different patients respond to different antivirals. For each treatment, there are data on what percentage of people respond: 20, 30, 40 percent, whatever. That information's out there, even for many experimental drugs.

Statistically, the likelihood that there is a drug that you'll respond to is greater than the probability of responding to any *one* drug. You must consider the universe of existing treatments, experimental and otherwise, and estimate the probability that you will respond to some drug or some combination of drugs. The odds are good. Therefore, you must get your doctor to try different treatments and different combinations of treatments. Be aggressive. When one doesn't work, recognize that and move on. Time is not on your side.

Don't expect doctors to think like this, however. First, they aren't trained to think statistically. They evaluate the potential benefits of each drug in isolation. That's bad statistical thinking. If I toss dice five times, I have a much higher probability of seeing snake eyes than if I toss them only once.

Second, both the hospital and your doctors have little to gain and lots to lose by hurrying. Even though they sincerely want to help you, they are by nature conservative — and their procedures are, too. They aren't good at recognizing when and how to switch people from one drug to another. If you keep in mind how their objectives and perspectives differ from yours, you'll negotiate more effectively with doctors, hospitals, and drug companies.

The FDA approved ddI in October 1991, two years after I started taking it. Any doctor can prescribe ddI now. But this story is repeating itself with other experimental drugs, right now. There are people who could use those drugs today, but can't get the bureaucracy to respond.

Here in Boston, I'm the ddI poster boy. When reporting the FDA approval of ddI, the local television stations chose to interview me and ... Doc Rayon! Now, I haven't told you this yet, but Rayon and I had been on the experimental drug merry-go-round before. In early 1987, after the chemotherapy I'd taken in the fall stopped working, I sought out Doc Rayon and asked her about AZT.

"Oh, no, it's too risky!" she exclaimed. Then she added, helpfully, "It hasn't been approved yet! It could do so much harm!"

In fact, AZT was in the middle of Phase Two studies. It became the treatment of choice for PWAs shortly thereafter.

Recently Doc Rayon was on the FDA panel that approved ddI by a 5-to-2 vote. On *her* TV interview, she stated that the FDA had lowered its standards by not dotting all the i's and crossing all the t's. She voted against approval. She's still snarling and harrumphing. Personally, I can't afford to wait until the children at the FDA learn penmanship.

Subsequently, Rayon was on the ddC panel. Again, she voted no. What do you think Doc Rayon's going to say about the *next* experimental drug?

At the end of *my* interview, the reporter asked if I had any final words. Well, I do!

1) I responded to ddI, *as I did to AZT*. My health stabilized, then improved. *I bought the right house.*

2) I was right about toxicities and ddI. At lower doses they're seeing little pancreatitis or neuropathy. And the toxicities appear to be reversible, as was true of AZT. *It's a good neighborhood.*

3) If I had listened to the doctors, particularly Rayon, I'd be dead today. As it is, *everyone wants to move into my neighborhood!*

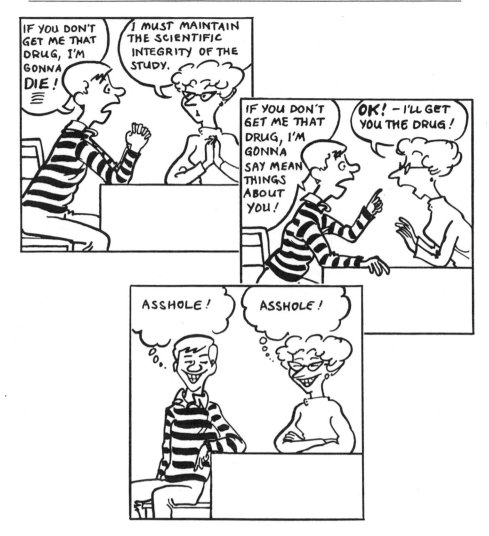

MORAL: **No one is Running the Show. It's up to you.**
You are the only one whose primary objective is to keep you alive.

OBTAINING EXPERIMENTAL DRUGS
Here's a worksheet for you to apply some of these concepts.

1. Remember a time you tried something new, non-routine, or experimental — maybe a product (cereal, software, pilot television program), or a service, or an activity.

The "experiment" was _____

Who was in charge? _____

Their objective was _____

My objective was _____

2. Do you know any people who have tried an experimental drug or therapy? Write their names here and the treatments.

3. Name an experimental treatment you would like to know more about.

4. Have you ever discussed experimental treatments with your doctor?

7

Reordering
Your Priorities

C an't a day go by without talk of AIDS?" Mario groused one day after I hung up the phone. A friend and I had been chatting about gas problems caused by ddI.

"It was just a phone call," I protested.

"It's the tip of an iceberg," he retorted. "Everything involves AIDS: work, friends, hobbies. You lack balance. And I'm sick of it."

I had to admit, my friend and I must have sounded like two grandpas talking about their bowel habits. You see, although I look reasonably healthy, my body isn't the body of a 42-year-old. It's more like that of a 70-year-old man. Like a 70-year-old, I may live thirty more years — if there is a cure for HIV. I still have my pre-HIV interests and personality, but my priorities are those of an old man. My friends and I talk about finances, insurance, and volunteer activities. We have weird ailments and joke about death, as long as it doesn't strike too close to home, which happens often enough. *I'm a gay senior citizen on rollerblades — flirting with college boys.*

If you're going to have a life — whether with HIV or with old age — you must learn to constructively adapt to changes and move on. There are some differences, however. Old people don't announce, "I've become old." People with HIV, on the other hand, frequently find that their condition is invisible until they announce it.

As you think about life with HIV, you may be asking yourself the following questions:

- Will I be isolated by and from friends who are HIV-negative? (Will I isolate myself?)
- How will I deal with medical and financial paperwork?

- What if I don't want to work full-time? Or at all?
- If I apply for disability, am I just giving up?
- Do you have to be sick to get disability?
- What if I have to work?
- How will I deal with friends who are HIV-positive?
- Can I keep HIV from taking over my life?

COPING WITH PROFOUND CHANGE

HIV affects your life dramatically. Many people become so focused on health care and the present that they lose their sense of the future. That's just for starters. HIV also has a way of creeping into every aspect of life: family, friendships, career interests, and hobbies.

Even old people, who've had decades to prepare for inevitable changes, have trouble coping. The prospect of so many changes layered over every part of your life is more than most of us want to face. So we try denial. In my own case, whether I wanted to face HIV or not, I had to. Shortly after I was diagnosed, KS began running amok on my legs and I had trouble walking.

But what if there is no health crisis? How do you start coping with profound change when you aren't forced to? Many people find that the invisibility of HIV makes it particularly difficult.

Unlike me, my friend Rachel learned she was HIV-positive through a routine blood test. There were no outer signs. Although she was "healthy" when she learned she was HIV-positive, her response was to cry, drink, and work hard. She isolated herself for several months, not even telling her husband.

On the surface, Rachel and I differ in many aspects. She is straight, married, a mother — and asymptomatic. Because she discovered her HIV status recently, she has made decisions in a society that is more knowledgeable and more supportive of HIV-positive people than when I started this adventure in 1986. In many ways, however, the HIV system has changed little. We are working the same system and dealing with similar issues, particularly this one: *How do you keep on LIVING with HIV?*

There is no right answer to this question. You need to hear several approaches and choose the pieces that might apply to you. Rachel is someone I learn from myself, so I've included her story here.

On Wednesday, April 25, 1990, I received a registered letter from the Red Cross, telling me not to donate any more blood and please call. I called immediately and was scheduled to see a social worker that afternoon.

I was shaken. I'd been giving blood regularly for years — most recently in January and then again in April — and never had a problem. If it were hepatitis, I thought, they would just tell me. The only other thing I could think of was HIV. But how could it be HIV? I didn't think I was at risk. Since 1983, I had been with only three men: my ex-lover Jack, my husband Albert, and a one-night stand after a Christmas party in 1989. In the front seat of a car. In a parking garage.

Besides, I had donated blood in January — no problem.

I drove alone to the local Red Cross. It was my day off. I had recently started a part-time contract at AIDS Action, organizing a conference for AIDS service providers in New England. Two months before, I had been laid off from a part-time public relations job at a computer company.

The Red Cross receptionist directed me to a small office. As I took my seat, the social worker waited quietly.

"Do you have any idea why you're being asked to come in here?" she began.

"I think you're going to tell me I'm HIV-positive."

"Is there any reason why you should think that?"

"No."

I swear she had a little smirk on her face.

Fuck you, bitch, I thought.

She told me I was positive — they'd already tested my blood twice — that was the procedure. Positive on both tests. I was in shock. Maybe there had been a mistake. The procedure was to run the tests again. The social worker called in a nurse, who drew some blood. As she did, I thought, *They must have switched my blood with someone else's.*

The first test results would be back the next day. The second would take a bit longer. We agreed she could call me at home with the results. I looked forward to a week of hell.

The social worker began asking me about my sexual history — to document transmission, I guess. My husband and I were having marital problems and had not been intimate for a long time, so I didn't think it could be him. Considering that I had donated blood in January — and it tested negative — the social worker thought it had to be this guy in the car.

I wasn't thinking clearly. I just didn't want to think I was going to die because I had an interlude in a car.

As I drove home, I thought, I don't want to die from this and even more I don't want to live with this. I wanted to kill myself.

I called my former job-sharing partner, Jennifer, and told her. She was distraught and supportive. I asked if she wanted to take over my job at AIDS Action. I didn't think I'd go back. As it happened, her husband had just been told he would be transferred to Hong Kong. She was crushed and didn't want to leave me.

I also told my boss, David, who was quickly becoming a friend and mentor. I walked into his office and said, "David, I just found out I'm HIV-positive." Unfortunately, David was preoccupied with caring for his best friend and colleague, Larry, who was sick. He sent me to a new company which provided medical case management for people with HIV. They were very helpful, but that was not enough. I wanted David to take the HIV away.

I told no one else and started making plans to kill myself.

I would visit my parents in Kansas City and get Seconal that I knew my father kept. He's a physician. I planned to bring the pills back to Boston and get a room at the Ritz-Carlton. I also arranged to meet my ex-lover, Jack, who also lived in Kansas City. Then I hopped a plane to Kansas City.

First things first. I looked for the Seconals. No luck. When I couldn't find the Seconal, I fantasized slitting my wrists at the Ritz — and somehow warning people to be careful of my HIV-infected blood. I dropped the thought — it was too gruesome. Then I met Jack and told him I was positive. I was secretly hoping I'd gotten HIV from him. But he had tested negative a year before. He has a gay doctor who knew to test him. When I told him I was positive, he was retested. Negative again.

I returned to Boston, crazed.

For the rest of the month, all I thought about was my three-year-old, Sarah. What age would she be when I died? If I got those ten years people talked about, she would be thirteen. That would be a fucking disaster. Thirteen-year-olds hate their mothers. She'd really hate me if I got sick and died at that age. I was a wreck.

My husband and I had been distant from each other for several months. I wasn't ready to talk about this. I threw myself into planning the conference, which was now relevant to me in a way I never anticipated.

I cried my way through the summer — and I'm not a crier. Nobody knew except Jennifer, who was in Hong Kong, and Jack, and my boss David. I drank a bottle of wine every night. On my days off I sat at home, watching TV and fantasizing. I didn't tell my husband what was going on until July. As the summer wore on, he convinced my case manager that I was an alcoholic. She thought I should check into an alcohol rehab center. As a compromise, I started seeing a social worker at a local hospital.

The conference I was planning was scheduled for early September. It was a big success — six hundred AIDS professionals and volunteers from around New England. Afterwards I crashed. I was depressed and lonely. Finally I told both my counselor and my social worker, "I have to find someone else to talk to." For-tunately, the social worker knew of a newly formed HIV-positive women's group. The following week, I went to the group's second meeting.

Joleen, who started the group, greeted me. There were five of us.

Joleen had been symptomatic for years but no one took her seriously. Her doctor told her she had cancer-phobia. Three weeks before her wedding, she took an HIV test and it came back positive. As she left the examination room, the receptionist asked, "Was it going to be a big wedding?" Joleen never went back to that doctor.

The others were Susan, who's into astrology; Lori, who had lived in New York and was still very druggy; and Diane. Lori and Diane are both married to IV-drug users.

The group had invited speakers from a predominantly gay health center on the topic of safe sex. Two very nice women introduced themselves and began talking about safe sex for lesbians! I had trouble following. Which partner is infected? Who's going down on whom? Dental dams? Which? Whom? I concentrated, trying to apply this information to me, but I was frustrated. We all were.

The support group's format was to have the guest speaker in the first hour, followed by an hour of peer support. So my first group was about ... lesbian sex. Not a promising start. By the end of the meeting, however, I knew I'd come back. I felt a connection with Joleen and that was enough. I was desperate to talk with someone.

For the first few months, I came home from the group horribly depressed. Then I realized: It *is* depressing. This isn't what I really want to do at night — sit around talking about HIV with a group of women I have nothing in common with except HIV! I'd rather be out dancing!

Nonetheless, I have to say it's a great group. Their stories have been invaluable to me. I get good advice and I've learned — after a few mishaps — to check things out carefully and compare experiences with other people who have HIV.

At the end of January, I attended a five-day empowerment workshop for people with HIV, called the Insight Seminar. Ordinarily I would not consider something like this. Insight is an offshoot of EST and I avoid anything New Age like the plague. But it was marketed to people with HIV, so I said what the hell.

After the third evening, I had a long chat with myself at home.

"What has been going on here?" I asked myself. "For the last eight months I've walked around thinking, *I can't bear this.*" Organizing the conference took my mind off it a bit, but when the conference was over, I went into a tailspin.

What is it I can't bear?

I realized my burden wasn't the disease itself. I wasn't in any physical pain yet. It was guilt. My daughter was going to lose her mother because I screwed some guy in the front seat of a car.

Finally I said, "Jesus, what did I do that was so terrible? It's not a crime to have been unhappily married and want some excitement. I'm sorry it turned out this way, but I did not believe I was at risk in 1989." I would have said it's a hard disease to get. I thought it required doing things I was not doing. And I certainly didn't think I could contract HIV from a one-night stand.

"Well, I'm sorry," I said aloud to the empty room, "but I'm going to go on. And I won't continue to feel guilty. This is ridiculous."

That was a turning point for me — a milestone, after which my life began to improve. I began mobilizing: coming out to my friends and family, searching for a job with benefits, and thinking about the future. I slowly became friends with a man I met at the seminar. It was my first new friendship since HIV. I wrote my parents and told them. They were very supportive. Later, I told colleagues at AIDS Action that I was HIV-positive. I don't advertise it but I don't hide it either.

I'd go completely public but for the fact that my daughter is in kindergarten and 90 percent of her classmates' mothers would not allow them to come to my house if they found out. When she's older it will be a little easier to deal with. Plus, her friends will be more independent and able to figure out how to keep seeing her. In the meantime, I need to protect her.

■

As Rachel describes, coping with the news that you are HIV-positive is a life-changing experience.

Many of you are acquainted with Elizabeth Kubler-Ross's work on death and dying. Kubler-Ross theorizes that people deal with loss in stages. I find her framework illuminates responses to HIV as well. Many people first try denial. When that doesn't work, they get angry and blame themselves or others. We work through the changes step by step.

The following chart shows how I see these stages. Does it apply to you?

HIV-Positive Coming-Out Process

STAGE	ATTITUDE
Denial	Shingles is not necessarily HIV-related. I don't need to get tested.
Anger	I caught HIV because I was a whore, *or* Why me?
Bargaining	I'll register at the AIDS organization, but I don't need to go there.
Depression	Life sucks.
Acceptance	My life's not so bad, *or* I want a new job.

In a way, coping with HIV is also like coming out as a gay person. You assess what you have and what you want in the light of changes. How you spend your time and what you get out of it. You begin to look at work, neighborhood, and family differently; you learn a new vocabulary; and you may find your social network changing. Some people find their existing network comes through for them; others must build new ones.

David Aronstein, who wrote a master's thesis on the coming-out process of gay people, believes there is an additional stage: *Crashing Out.* At this point, newly "out" people live, eat, and breathe their gay identity. For some that means throwing themselves into dating or sex; for others it is political organizing. "I want all my friends to be gay."

A similar process may occur for HIV-positive people. Mario thinks I crashed out and took him with me.

ASSESSING YOUR LIFE

Given the changes HIV brings, you must assess your life: What still works and what does not?

Before HIV, you may or may not have visualized life as a bowl full of cherries. I find it useful to think of life after HIV as a bowl of T-cells. Some parts of life are satisfying and non-stressful: I imagine them giving me T-cells. Other aspects of life — the unsatisfying, stressful things — chew up T-cells. *Your job is to keep that bowl full.*

To do this, you must evaluate:
- which activities give you T-cells and which take them away; and
- whom you spend time with.

Let's start with the people in your life — your network.

To a certain extent, your network will adapt to HIV on its own. Once you come out, some people call more and some people call less. The supportive people in your life become more prominent. Sometimes, however, you must eliminate unsupportive people or stressful interactions. They cost you too many T-cells.

For example, it always bothered me that my mother did not accept my homosexuality. Before my AIDS diagnosis, I accepted her resistance as part of her mental illness. Afterwards, her homophobia became more virulent and harder to deal with. In the summer of 1987, when I was still weak from high doses of interferon, she lathered herself into a state and called me one day.

"I told you this would happen!" she shrieked.

"Told me what would happen?"

"This ... this AIDS!"

I called her less frequently after that. I came to think of each call as eating up T-cells.

In 1990, she asked, "When are you getting married again?"

"Mother, Mario and I have been living together thirteen years. I'm gay. I have AIDS! I am *not* getting married again. Ever!"

"But you dated girls in high school," she countered. "You even got married!"

"Mother, that was the sixties! We all did crazy things then!"

Fuming, I told Mario of this phone call. We debated whose parents were crazier.

"One thing is clear, Bob," he observed. "Talking to Babs is making *you* crazy."

He was right. After thinking it over for a couple days, I called back and said firmly, "Mom, my therapist told me not to talk to you. It's too stressful. Don't call me any more!"

I hung up, confident that she would not call. She took therapists very seriously.

My brother Stevie called shortly thereafter. "I didn't know you were seeing a therapist," he began. "Are you all right?"

"Oh," I admitted, "I stopped seeing my therapist months ago. I made that up so she would stop harassing me."

"I wish I'd thought of that!" he chuckled. "Her calls make Jean and me crazy, too! Good job, Robert!"

A couple months later, Stevie called and said, "Ma just called. She said you're doing well."

"Really? How would she know?"

"She saw you in the *Herald*. And again on TV, talking about drugs. She said you look wonderful!"

The *Boston Herald* had quoted me extensively in an article on ddI. A large grinning photo of me was included.

Stevie sighed. "It's a shame our family has to communicate through the media."

■

In addition to dropping people from your network, you can add new, positive people. Rachel, for example, joined a support group. I volunteered at an AIDS service organization. Other people adopt new hobbies or take out personal ads.

Positive steps like these require time and energy — and

changes in your priorities. This brings us to how you spend your time. Here's a diagram showing how an HIV-negative working adult might spend his time:

A TYPICAL LIFE BEFORE HIV

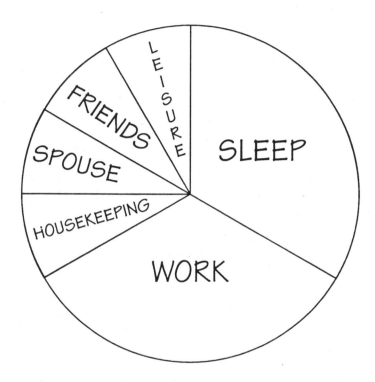

After HIV, you must somehow fit in new pieces:

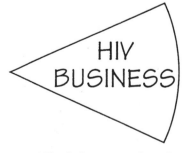

- Medical homework (Researching treatments)
- Insurance paperwork
- Getting support
- Giving support
- Medical appointments

All of this together I call **HIV Business.**

How will you fit the HIV Business piece into your life? This is the question that HIV-positive people get angry about, with good reason! Nobody asked for HIV. It threatens your income, destroys your health, shatters your future, and then demands that you spend time managing it.

In spite of your anger, you must face the question: Where will the time to manage HIV come from? What activities can you cut back? Stressful ones, I hope. For most of us, the big variables are job, leisure, spouse, sleep, and maybe house-keeping. As you visualize your own pie chart, do you see activities you'd like to spend more time on? Or things you'd like to cut out?

Too many people think they can steal the time needed for HIV Business from their sleep time or from activities they cherish, like time with friends or spouse. That is very short-term thinking. You need to invest in your life, not steal from it.

Use the worksheet below to estimate how much time you'll need or want to spend on HIV in a typical month. Then take another look at the pie chart and think about where this time could come from.

HIV BUSINESS WORKSHEET

For each activity, estimate the hours you need to spend per month. Consider your life as it is today.

Activity	Hours Per Month (est.)
Doctor appointments (including travel to and from)	_____
Medical homework (reading and calls)	_____
Insurance paperwork	_____
Providing support to HIV+ friends	_____
Dealing with your family's anxiety... telephone calls, etc.	_____
Therapy appointments	_____
Support group	_____
Making new friends	_____
Going to the drugstore	_____
HIV/AIDS fundraisers	_____
Extra sleep	_____
Extra rest	_____
Other	_____
TOTAL TIME:	_____

You probably lost fifty T-cells just filling out this worksheet. Read the next section to get them back!

MAKING ROOM FOR HIV BUSINESS

Making room means rearranging. At the risk of over-simplifying, there are three areas you can rearrange to make room for HIV Business:

1) where you live;
2) your work life; and
3) your relationships.

People relocate for many reasons: to be closer to work or medical care, to get away from a stressful environment, or to be less isolated. I moved from the country to the city. Others do the opposite. Some people begin living with roommates, others decide to live alone. I'm sure you can think of other examples.

Here are some cases of people I know who renegotiated their relationship with work:

• Larry restructured his job at AIDS Action, restricting the number of projects and hours and the kinds of issues he dealt with. "I'm just the finance director now," he said once, "and I like it. I focus on my own department. It works and I go home."

• Joe, a self-employed masseur, had no disability insurance and no way to obtain any once he was symptomatic. He needed to keep working. Joe cut back on his volunteer projects, so he'd have more energy for his massage practice. He used some of this freed-up time to write theater reviews for a local paper.

• Michael Connolly's lover, also named Michael, was a purchasing manager for a chain of gourmet stores. He was able to persuade his boss to hire a part-time assistant so he could cut back to a four-day week. He used Wednesdays for doctor visits and HIV paperwork and to start a garden that became his passion.

• Elliot ended a relationship, moved to San Francisco, and ultimately switched careers. He dumped computers and went back to school for interior design. The last I heard, he was dating a bodybuilder he called Muffy.

■

Another way to renegotiate your work life is to get on disability. I'm a strong proponent of disability insurance. I continued working at Yankee for a year after my diagnosis and avoided disability because I thought, *Going on disability means you're giving up.*

As work got less interesting and more stressful, I reconsidered. I knew that treatment and HIV Business would continue taking up a lot of time. I was stealing that time from work, where I was absent a lot. In part, I was also short-changing other things I wanted to spend time on: Mario, friends, and hobbies. With mixed feelings, I finally decided to apply for disability.

"Am I giving up?" I wondered. Within three months, my outlook changed. *Disability wasn't so bad.* It provides me a steady, although reduced income. I'm lucky in that I have a good disability income and my lover has a good job. Most important, disability allowed me to fit HIV Business into my life, without wrecking it. I have time to enjoy the spontaneity of the day. I have continued my career by volunteering and I get the rest, sleep, and relaxation I need. I also got to write a book.

Most people I know who get on disability find their health improves once they're free of the stress of working full-time and scrambling to fit everything in. This is not something to rush into, since there are others who find themselves depressed and isolated by the loss of structure that work provides.

Once you realize that you might like to work less someday — even if you're not sick — fringe benefits become a higher priority. Unlike me, but like many people with HIV, Rachel realized her situation was not ideal. Consequently, she had a large piece of homework to do. Here's her account:

> Talking to my support group members, I realized I wanted as much independence and control over my life as possible. I wanted to spend time with my daughter — and saw that this depended on having secure insurances, in particular, health insurance I could take with me if I chose to work part-time, *before* having health problems. Obtaining benefits became a consuming passion.
>
> I couldn't use my husband's health insurance because his company, a small family business, feared

losing their health insurance policy and would probably fire him if they knew I was HIV-infected. I was working as a temporary employee, on contract, so I was not eligible for AIDS Action's group insurance or disability. Under COBRA, I had the right to continue my group insurance (Aetna) from my previous employer, for eighteen months. It was a lousy policy, however. Were I to convert to an individual policy after eighteen months, for example, my medical coverage would be capped at $10,000 — the equivalent of a one-week stay in the hospital!

Bob told me the solution was to get a job with good group health, disability, and life insurance policies. I started looking. I decided the benefits were primary and the salary was secondary. I liked working around people who were aware of HIV so I focused on hospitals and universities.

While job hunting, I managed to get individual life insurance. I also tried to keep everything out of the Medical Information Bureau database. I paid my doctors and social worker out of pocket — and filed no claims on my insurance.

In March, I accepted a fundraising contract at AIDS Action, gambling that it would lead to a permanent job. It did. When I started full-time in the summer, I got some very bad advice about insurance.

I was offered a choice of health plans: an HMO (Bay State) and an indemnity carrier (Lincoln). The benefits manager told me I could not convert the HMO policy to individual coverage if I left or went part-time. But he was wrong. The only problem was that my medication would no longer be covered if I switched from group to individual.

Based on that advice, I went with Lincoln, the indemnity carrier. In fact, the benefits manager had it backwards. The HMO offered what I needed: portability and high coverage limits. Lincoln had the same cap as my Aetna policy $10,000 limit if you convert from group to individual! And Bay State did not! Most importantly, Lincoln had a twelve-month pre-existing condition exclusionary clause, whereas Bay State had none. When I realized all this and asked to switch to the HMO, I found I had to wait until their open enrollment period, almost a year later! It was grotesque.

I've come to realize that benefits people are no better or worse than doctors. They're not perfect. Even more so in an AIDS organization, where staff are trained on the job and we're all improvising and learning as we go along. I assumed this manager knew best because this was an AIDS organization and I wasn't the first person with HIV he'd met.

I learned a valuable lesson, namely, that I didn't know the extent of my assumptions and of my own ignorance. I didn't know all the questions to ask. That's why you rely on people who've been in the same situation, as I do now in my support group.

■

Finally, you might find you need to renegotiate relationships, too, particularly with your spouse or lover. Needs, resources, energy, priorities — when any one of these changes, arrangements that worked before HIV may no longer be optimal.

Mario and I have always lived very independent lives. Once we moved into Boston and I cut back on my volunteer work, we thought we would enjoy our time together more. After thirteen years living together, this was harder than we expected. For a while we blamed each other's attitudes. I worried that Mario was isolated and had too few gay friends. He objected to my all-consuming HIV activism. In the spring of 1991, we began couples counseling.

In weekly sessions, which often included homework, Andre taught us to communicate clearly what we wanted and didn't want. We talked about what bothers us; how we think; how we make each other crazy. In particular, we worked on treating each other in special ways. Since we both feel displaced at times by HIV, this was important.

A week after Christmas, Andre asked what gifts we'd exchanged. We rattled off a half-dozen presents each. Shirts, coffee mugs, kitchen gadgets, tickets to *Les Miserables*, a *Fantasia* video, and more.

As we finished the session, Mario asked Andre, "What did you and your lover get each other?"

"Well, I flew my parents in from the Midwest, which was

expensive. So Rufus and I decided to buy ourselves one big present this year."

I had been only half listening to this exchange, as I idly studied a flower arrangement on the glass coffee table and wondered how many hours Andre had spent getting the seven flowers just so. Now my curiosity was piqued. One big present?

"What was that?" asked Mario.

"A juicer."

"Oh, that's very nice," said Mario, in the same tone he used when Jean told him there was a spirit sitting on his shoulder. ("Is it a good spirit or a bad spirit?" he asked, looking at his shoulder. "A good spirit," she replied. "That's nice," he said, continuing with his meal.)

In the hallway afterwards Mario said, "Do you believe that, Bob? A juicer?! Andre's as crazy as the rest of them."

"He's actually pretty sane for a mental health professional," I countered.

But we had met our objectives and stopped counseling soon thereafter. Although we stopped therapy, we still work on the issues Andre identified. I am more likely to decline media invitations, lobbying opportunities, and fundraising commitments. And Mario joins me more often when I do participate. I can't say we've fixed all the imbalances in our lives, but we are more aware of them. Consequently, when tempted to start hurling knives at each other, we are more able to listen, imagine some solutions, and compromise.

CLEANING THE HIV LITTER BOX

Once you have major HIV Business out of the way, insurances, a will, and so on things calm down. However, if you go on disability or see the doctor frequently, your mailbox soon becomes a litter box. Disability insurance generates detailed correspondence which requires attention. And hospital bills are almost always screwed up. According to the February 1990 issue of *Money* magazine, 90 percent of all hospital bills contain errors. If you monitor these bureaucratic details as you do your health, you can prevent crises that stress you out and blow your T-cells. The rule is:

When the bureaucracy tosses you a curve ball, don't panic.

Don't take responsibility for fixing the problem. Adopt a more realistic and less stressful goal — one that chews up no T-cells. That goal is: *Keep the ball in their court.* Achieving this can be surprisingly easy and low stress: *Whenever the ball comes your way, bounce it back to them.*

Here's an example. I've been playing ball with Beth Israel over erroneous bills since 1988. I have not received *a single* correct bill since then.

I have two insurance policies:

1) a Blue Cross Blue Shield Master Medical policy from my previous employer. It pays for most things and costs me nothing (my employer pays 100 percent); and

2) a Medicare policy, which I am eligible for because I receive SSDI. It pays for anything left over and costs me $40 a month.

Since I started taking ddI and recovered my health, I have two regular monthly appointments — one with Millie and one to receive aerosolized pentamidine. Nonetheless, every month, I get a ten-page, computer-generated bill containing erroneous charges dating back to 1989.

I figured out the problem years ago. If correctly done, my Blue Cross Blue Shield should be billed first, then Medicare should be billed for the remainder. For example, on a $300 bill, BCBS should pay $275 — the other $25 being my copayment, which Medicare should pay.

Unfortunately, the hospital frequently bills Medicare first and gets rejected. Medicare will not pay until BCBS has paid its portion. When Medicare rejects the bill, the hospital then tries to bill me. That's the major problem. The minor one is that the hospital sometimes takes more than a year to finally bill BCBS. And BCBS refuses to pay bills not submitted within twelve months. Guess who the hospital sends the bill to then?

When I first contacted the hospital billing department, in 1988, a representative blamed the computer.

"Fine," I said, "but you do understand that between my two policies, everything is paid for?"

"Yes, I see."

"And you understand that you must bill Blue Cross first?" He did.

I wrote a letter confirming this and called periodically thereafter. The erroneous bills got larger and more complicated — and my account was eventually referred to a collection agency, which sent me a letter. This irked me, since a bad credit report can prevent me from getting a mortgage, among other things. I realized this was an opportunity, however. Submitting a false credit report is a punishable offense. I could sue Beth Israel for damages, although I had no intentions of doing so. Here are the letters. (Mine was originally handwritten. I've retyped it for this book.)

ROBERT RIMER   NOVEMBER 12, 1988
199 VAUGHN HILL RD.
BOLTON, MA 01740
                      RE:
                      Patient Name: RIMER, ROBERT
                      Acct. No: 382724

Dear Mr/Ms RIMER:
    The Beth Israel Hospital has consulted us
concerning your overdue balance of $194.10 for
services beginning 07/12/88.
    We feel our client has been considerate and
lenient in handling your account, therefore,
this letter is to advise you that your account
will be placed in our collection department for
examination and appropriate action, unless the
Beth Israel Hospital Ambulatory Department, BR-
308, 330 Brookline Avenue, Boston, MA 02215,
receives payment in full directly from you
within ten (10) days.
    If you have already mailed your payment,
thank you, and please disregard this notice.
    Free Care, Public Assistance and Payment
Plans are available to financially qualified per-
sons. Please contact (617) 735-3441 for further
information.
                      Sincerely,

                      B. Irving
                      Medical Audit systems
                      Division of Walker Associates

TO: B. IRVING — WALKER ASSOCIATES 12/4/88
FR: ROBERT RIMER 38 27 24

I am incensed that this matter is still un-
resolved. The letter you sent me is insulting
and inappropriate.

The overdue balance of $194.10 is incorrect,
021858919, chemotherapy, administered by a nurse
is covered by BC/BS at 100% You can see by the
attached BI bill summary that other charges for
$194.10 were paid by BC/BS.

THERE IS A CODING ERROR AT THE BI

I have spoken, since July, at least once a month
to Maria, Janice & others when I called the billing inquiry number. I have personally spoken to
PAUL BAKER, 3 or 4 times last month, who assured
me the problem has been found and he personally
said he would handle the matter.

I am sick (AIDS diagnosis 3/86) and cannot be
bothered with this. I have spent approximately
$20 in phone charges trying to resolve this mat-
ter.

The incompetance [*sic*] of the administrative
staff at the BI is mind-boggling.

If this matter is not resolved immediately, I
will seek legal recourse for this harrassment
[*sic*].

PLEASE RESPOND IN WRITING

Attachments
cc: DIRECTOR — BI HOSPITAL ABULATORY [*sic*] DEPT
      PAUL BAKER

                        ROBERT RIMER
                        [PHONE NUMBER]

As you can see, I did *not* make my letter nice and neat — and you don't have to either! I'm not Miss Manners. I'm a PWA who doesn't want to lose T-cells on hospital incompetence.

The hospital called off the collection agency at that point, although the problems remained uncorrected. Six months later, our ball game entered a new phase. The billing clerk explained that BI was installing a new computer system which would handle the problem. It would take a year. Since then I've spoken to a series of hapless clerks and their supervisors — *and never paid the bill.*

I always note the name of the clerk I'm talking to, record the date, and write down what that person agrees to do and by when. Then I politely ask for the supervisor's name, title, and mailing address — "just in case the problem doesn't get corrected."

Sometimes they ask *me* to fix the problem, e.g., by calling Blue Cross Blue Shield! In these cases, I say, "I've had AIDS for (four, five, six) years. I'm really not well enough to deal with this — and I'm not supposed to. Please let me speak with your supervisor."

When I get the supervisor, I tell him the whole story. Most importantly, I don't worry and I don't get upset. I chat, laugh, and joke, pretending I have all the time and patience in the world. And I make it clear that I am not paying.

Patience is required, because you are often dealing with new staff and must therefore start from the very beginning. If you expect the bureaucracy to lose everything and have absolutely no memory, you will be less frustrated.

Here's another example. Around Thanksgiving of 1991, it was time for my quarterly call to the hospital billing department. Rick answered.

A new one, I thought. I told him I had been treated for AIDS at Beth Israel since 1986. He clucked sympathetically. Somewhere in the process, he concluded I was gay and alluded to boyfriend problems. We commiserated briefly. Then I described the billing problem.

"It is impossible for me to owe anything. You are not submitting the bills correctly to Blue Cross and Medicare."

I told him there were numerous entries on my bill saying "Claim Rejected by Medicare." My theory? The hospital was billing Medicare first, instead of Blue Cross.

As we finished up, he said, "The new computer system has been in place for a while and it's all debugged. I can't believe your problem hasn't been fixed."

"I'll bet it's worse next month!" I said brightly.

"No, no, I'll look into it right away," he assured me.

I thanked him, made a note in my file — and made a one-dollar bet with Michael that the next bill would be worse.

To give the system a chance, we waited for the second bill. Two months. When it arrived I ripped open the envelope with relish, saying, "I'm gonna win a dollar!" Pages of gobbledygook.

I turned on my speaker phone so that Michael could listen, and called Rick in billing.

"Rick, you told me this would be fixed. It's not fixed!"

"You must have spoken with someone else."

"Oh no, I have it noted right here that I spoke with you. We discussed our boyfriends. Don't you remember?"

There was a pause. "Oh, yes. I remember now." He assured me again the problem would be corrected.

"R-e-a-l-l-y? That would be awfully nice, but frankly I'm doubtful. This has been going on for three years. Would you like me to read you some of the correspondence?"

"No, that's not necessary. Every time you call we note it on the computer."

"Must be quite a file!"

He grunted.

I continued. "What do you think the problem is?"

Rick made a guess. He did not remember my explanation from the previous conversation. I went over it again. We concluded with more promises.

After a couple more erroneous bills, I called again. A supervisor told me Rick was no longer there. I summarized the story for her. She responded sympathetically and said she had been transferred into billing to help "clean it up."

"Where's Rick?" I asked.

"I'm afraid he's not here any more." She lowered her voice. "He was the most incompetent one we've ever had!"

"We could debate that a bit..."

We chatted some more.

"Medicare is denying payment because they say — correctly — that I have other insurance as my primary carrier."

She agreed — and suggested that I call Medicare.

I hooted. "I'm sure I'll have lots of luck with Medicare! Seriously, the problem is between your computer and Medicare's. I can't fix that for you. Have your computer people call Medicare!"

She made the usual promises and we finished up amicably. A month later, I received another screwed-up bill. I added it to my billing file, which is eighteen inches thick. I don't expect them ever to get it all straightened out. For my own peace of mind, I attached documentation to my will, so the executor of my estate will know not to pay these bills if, by some quirk, I'm not here someday.

In your new career as an HIV-positive person, you will encounter numerous snafus. They come with the territory. You need to make time for them but also to adopt a healthy attitude.

When errors occur, promptly contact the agency responsible and tell them what the problem is. Don't blame the people you speak with. It's probably not their fault. Let them know why you think there is a problem, simply and directly. Ask how they plan to investigate and fix it. Be clear that it is their problem. Wish them luck. Keep records.

And Play Ball!

PLAYING BALL, PART ONE: SUPPORTING FRIENDS

Earlier, I said that giving and getting support are part of HIV Business. Occasionally, more than support is needed. Sometimes friends need active care and assistance. As well as a chance to help a friend, this is also an opportunity to learn more about HIV bureaucracies. Here's what happened when Larry needed home health care.

It was May 1990. Larry had left AIDS Action on full-time disability nine months earlier. Now he was getting sick. He lived in a four-story walk-up in a transitional neighborhood. He began having trouble walking up stairs — and had fallen in the shower a couple times. He got easily confused. Soon it was clear to Larry and his friends that we needed to plan for his care.

One evening, a dozen friends gathered at my apartment to discuss with Larry how we would care for him. Larry wanted to live as normal a life as possible, in his own space. We agreed to stay overnight with him and visit often. We also began looking for an apartment in a building with an elevator and a ramp.

In late May, Larry was hospitalized with kidney stones, a side effect of his toxoplasmosis medication. While in the hospital, he became incontinent.

"If I can't control my bowels, what can I control?" he asked as Michael massaged his feet one night.

"Us," Michael replied. "You can let us know when to talk and when to be quiet and what feels good to you."

Larry sighed. Depressed, he withdrew into himself for hours at a time.

Numerous doctors examined him for neurological symptoms. The exams followed a simple script: "Point to me ... Now touch your nose ... What year is it? ... Who is president?" When a doctor entered the room, Larry would roll his eyes and touch his nose with a grand flourish.

Upon his release, Larry stabilized briefly, then had increasing memory problems — and trouble moving his left arm. The doctor recommended a brain biopsy. Maybe something treatable would be found. There seemed to be no other options, so he consented and was hospitalized again.

The biopsy was inconclusive. Larry recovered in the hospital for a couple weeks. He used a wheelchair and rarely spoke in sentences. David and I were visiting him one afternoon when a resident stopped by for a neurological exam. Larry had not spoken all afternoon and we were feeling glum.

After the pointing was done, the doctor asked the year. "1990."

"And who is the president of the United States?"

Larry looked at the doctor and then at us, eyes twinkling. "John Waters."

We erupted at the name of Larry's favorite — and quite demented — film director. Whatever the doctor may have scribbled in response, we knew Larry was telling us not to worry.

In the meantime, we had found an appropriate apartment in a conveniently located building and we transferred Larry's belongings. After he got out of the hospital, I scheduled friends overnight and during the day, but it was difficult. All Larry's friends were working full-time except for me.

His case manager had already contacted the insurance company and requested home care, which proved to be a struggle. Larry's insurance policy covered "skilled nursing care" at home, but not custodial home care. The focus had to be administering medications and monitoring his health. Laundry, shopping, housework, changing diapers, and bathing him were not, in themselves, needs sufficient to justify home care.

The bottom line is that when someone is failing and unable to live alone safely, there are three options:

1) Stay in the hospital, which costs the insurance company thousands of dollars per day.

2) Go to a residential hospice, where the intent is not to treat you, but to keep you comfortable. This costs about $400 a day.

3) Obtain home care, which now costs about $400 a day for 16-hour coverage, and $600 a day for round-the-clock coverage.

Choosing between these options is not a private matter between you and your doctor. An insurance company "case manager" has final say. Insurance companies assign a "case manager" to any person with an expensive illness, including people with HIV. These insurance company employees are *cost control managers*. They rarely meet patients and often have no medical training. They decide if you will receive home care or not.

The cost control manager approved eight hours of care, five days a week. We contacted the local hospice organization, which assigned a nurse to Larry and subcontracted the actual care to a nationwide temp agency called Olsten, which sent us the home health assistant. (Talk about moving parts!)

David was at Larry's to greet and orient the home health aide, a middle-aged woman. After chatting a bit, David asked, "Have you lifted patients out of bed before?"

Yes, she had.

"Have you taken care of an AIDS patient before?"

Startled, she said, "I'm sorry, I don't do that!"

David excused himself and called the hospice agency, which promised to send someone else the next day.

"That's fine," he said. "I'll put this woman on the phone now and you can send her home."

"She'll just leave at the end of her shift," the nurse told him.

"Please get her out now," said David and they did. Afterwards, he called me. Our confidence in hospice management had evaporated.

Emmanuel arrived the next day — a tall black Panamanian who spoke flawless English. He seemed gay, but offered no details about himself except that he was a Buddhist — the kind that chants. Emmanuel was always in conflict with Olsten about his paycheck, how much he was getting paid. Once he didn't show up because the check had not been ready for him the previous day. He was also late a lot, which caused those who stayed overnight to be late for work and all of us to worry.

Nonetheless, Larry seemed happy around Emmanuel. Emmanuel got him out of bed and into the shower and took him outdoors in nice weather. After a week, I realized our friends couldn't cover afternoons and evenings and do overnights, too. We needed more coverage. As required by the insurance company, both Larry's primary care physician and a hospice nurse documented Larry's need for 24-hour coverage.

Larry's private case manager called the insurance company first, without success. The woman at the insurance company kept saying no.

Then I called. I prepared by reminding myself first that the cost control manager was not our enemy and was only doing a job. My approach was to make her more of an ally. To do so, I would try two appeals — first to her humanity, by talking about Larry, his wishes, and his friends. More importantly, I would keep our differing objectives in mind. Her job was to minimize cost.

I started off simply, "We're trying real hard to take care of Larry. I just don't know what to do. His doctor says he needs to be in the hospital. But Larry really doesn't want to go die in the hospital." Of course, I knew the cost control manager did not want Larry in the hospital either. That was the most expensive solution.

I explained the logistics of evening and overnight coverage, laundry, meals, and so forth. We spent twenty minutes discussing the people who were pitching in and what each of us could do. I purposefully spent a long time on this. I didn't want her to think phone calls with me would be cheap or easy.

"Why can't *you* do it?" she asked repeatedly.

Finally I said, "I'm trying to help him, but frankly, I have AIDS myself."

She fell silent. Then she authorized two shifts a day, morning and afternoon, seven days a week.

We had agreed on the objective of keeping Larry out of the hospital, because I convinced her that it was an imminent possibility. I had gotten the system to give us the staff we needed. Now I turned my thoughts to managing them.

PLAYING BALL, PART TWO: WATCHING OUT FOR THIEVES

On crankier days, I refer to the bureaucrats who fill up my mailbox as goons. As you know, I'm prepared for goons. Sometimes I even enjoy dealing with them! (I call it sport.) I was surprised to learn the bureaucrats sometimes send you thieves, however. I was not originally prepared for that, now I know better.

The hospice sent us two more home health aides — John for weekends and Floyd for afternoons.

Larry was deteriorating and could not communicate easily. I wanted to be sure the aides would go beyond the letter of their job and truly care for him. In particular, should there be any problem, David and I were adamant that the home health aide reach one of us.

I was there to greet and orient them: laundry, keys, how the bed works, the medications, how to reach friends and family, and so on. I wanted to establish rapport and set expectations from the outset. I wanted them to know I was actively monitoring Larry's care and might pop in at any time.

John was tall, blond, and approaching middle age. He had a gentle, frumpy look. After introducing him to Larry and showing him the apartment, I sat him in the living room to chat. It was an interview, really. You remember those from chapter 5.

"Do you live around here?"

"Yes, just outside the city."

"Are you married?"

"Yes."

"Any children?"

"Yes, two kids, a boy and a girl."

"That's nice. But it must be inconvenient for you to come into town."

"Not really. Besides," he offered, "I like to go to Jacques [a nearby transvestite bar] for a nightcap. Sometimes I stop by one of the other gay bars."

He tells the truth, I said to myself. *Good. I'll think about the transvestite part later...*

"Do you like your job?"

"Yes, I do." He told me about previous patients with some fondness.

I may not have to check up on him that much, I thought.

John worked weekends, from 7:00 a.m. to 11:00 p.m. He was on time and reliable. He came when he said he would. He was also the most skilled in getting Larry out of bed and in and out of his wheelchair.

Floyd worked the afternoon and evening shift. A wiry, energetic man, straightforwardly gay, unlike the other two, Floyd explained that he had a second job, as a live-in aide to an older, disabled man. He turned out to be unreliable. Over the next three weeks his lunch breaks ballooned from twenty minutes to two hours. He also came in late and tried to leave early.

Because Larry was incontinent, there was a lot of laundry, which I oversaw. A few days after Floyd started, I brought in $50 in quarters. The next afternoon, they were all gone. I called David, upset.

"A funny thing happened, David. All the quarters are gone!"

"Oh, Bob," he replied, "you're worrying about quarters!"

"Well, it's not just the money. I have to go get more quarters, for one thing. And what else are they doing if they're taking quarters? What are they doing to Larry?"

I confronted Emmanuel and Floyd the next afternoon, when their shifts overlapped. I thought it was Emmanuel.

"Gee, that was an awful lot of laundry that you guys did," I began.

"Sure was," agreed Emmanuel. "I did four or five loads."

"And you, Floyd?"

"I did a bunch, too. At least that many."

"That's funny," I said. "Even if it's ten loads between you, that's only $20. Did you misplace the other quarters? There was $50 worth."

Emmanuel wrinkled his forehead and looked down his glasses at me, annoyed. "Please don't accuse me of stealing quarters. I'm not stealing quarters."

As Emmanuel prepared to leave, Floyd shook his shoulders indignantly. "How dare you accuse me of stealing quarters!" he harrumphed.

"Maybe I'm mistaken," I said, looking him in the eye. "Here are some more." The rate of quarter theft dropped thereafter.

"Just how many quarters are they allowed to steal a week?" I asked David one day. He groaned. At the same time, I scooped up Larry's credit cards and checkbooks, for safekeeping.

I began to have doubts about Floyd. Not so much his tardiness or excessive lunch breaks as the fact that he lied about them, apparently not knowing that Larry's friends talked to each other. For example, Floyd asked Michael, who was staying overnight, to relieve him early, "because I didn't get my lunch break today." The second time this happened, Michael asked me why Floyd wasn't getting lunch breaks — and learned that Floyd's breaks were running two hours long.

One day Floyd failed to show up altogether. Olsten replaced him with an inexperienced twenty-year-old. As Larry grew weaker, we knew he needed more than home health coverage. On Monday, July 16, my fortieth birthday, I accompanied Larry in an ambulance to Boston's AIDS hospice. He died four days later.

In early August, when Larry's bank statement arrived, I was surprised to find two canceled checks, totaling over $3000, written to charities in Rhode Island. The handwriting was not Larry's. And a couple calls to Rhode Island established that no such charities existed. Earlier in the month, a friend of Larry's had reported a check missing after an early-evening visit. Now her bank statement arrived — showing an $800 bogus check.

I filed a report with the Boston police. Then I called the hospice agency director, who said he was appalled.

"What can we do?" he asked.

"You can reimburse us!"

"I think you should try to get the bank to reimburse you, first."

I called the bank. They said to speak with Olsten. I called

Olsten, where a manager claimed the hospice agency was responsible for reimbursing us. (Here we go again! These guys have played ball before!) I asked for her boss, the agency director, whom I told about the theft of checks. She said Olsten had recently received a similar complaint from another client to whom Floyd had been assigned — she had dismissed Floyd without filing charges.

"Don't you check for criminal records when you hire someone?" I asked.

"We used to, but that was too expensive."

"How do we know he's not out there working for a competitor of yours right now?"

She had no answer to that one.

Meanwhile, no word from the police. I left messages. The officer in charge was out for a few days. Floyd, however, left a message on Michael's answering machine. He'd left a shirt at Larry's and would like it back! This seemed curious — and bold.

Michael called me and said, "You've met your match. You can't work this system! Not as well as Floyd, anyway."

"It's not over till it's over," I replied, and called the police again. This time the officer was there.

"We simply don't know where this Floyd is," he said.

Michael left his office and came over to my house. We went to work — Sherlock Holmes and Watson! We had a phone number, but no address. First we checked the phone book. Floyd wasn't listed. We called the number we had. Floyd answered. We hung up, flabbergasted, and called the police.

"We have Floyd's phone number and he's at home right now. Go arrest him."

"We still need an address."

"Can't you just call the telephone company and get the address? You are the police department, after all."

"No, we can't do that. The phone company doesn't allow it." (More moving parts.)

"But there's another complaint filed against Floyd with his last employer! We just confirmed that! He steals from sick people!"

"I'm sorry, but we have no record of that complaint."

"That's because it was outside of Boston! Call Newton!"

"Well, I'm very busy. And we still need an address to arrest someone."

Michael and I decided to track Floyd down. What would Columbo do? We considered inviting Floyd over to Larry's apartment to retrieve his shirt, then locking him in and calling the police. That seemed risky. We needed another option.

What would Perry Mason and Paul Drake do? They'd head over to Floyd's last known address. Everything came back to the address. Who had an address for Floyd?

We called the temp agency, Olsten, again. The director checked Floyd's job application, which was several years old. The phone number matched. She gave us the address. A lead!

Michael and I drove downtown and parked near a low, block-long apartment building — the address recorded in the Olsten files. There were no names on the buzzers or the mailboxes. We peeked in the windows, then walked around back, looking for trash that might have Floyd's name on it. No luck. No clues.

Stymied, we walked over to AIDS Action, a few blocks away. As we were chatting in the mailroom about our new careers as private eyes a staffer heard us tittering about Floyd and said, "That name sounds familiar. I think we got a call from him!"

We ran down to her office.

"Yes," she said, "a Floyd called and inquired about volunteering with PWAs. Said he would like to help around the house."

We erupted. "Yes, Floyd finds working with PWAs most *rewarding.*"

Unfortunately, she had already forwarded a volunteer application to him and discarded the message. Until he responded, there would be no record of his address. He never did respond. In the end, Larry's estate was never reimbursed. Too many moving parts!

On the one hand, I was furious. We had trusted Floyd to take care of Larry and he had violated that trust. On the other hand, I had to admit that Floyd certainly knew how to work a system — even better than I! As far as we know, Floyd's still on the loose.

Don't misunderstand me. Home health care is a valuable service, when all else fails. But understand what to expect. You — or your friends — will end up with strangers in your home, who will be "managed" from a distance. As with doctors, you'll get better service and find life easier if you find time to interview your home health aides, set expectations clearly, and motivate them to take initiative.

That night, I recounted our adventure to Mario. "Larry would have been proud of us," I glowed. "We were like Perry Mason and Della Street."

"More like Lucy and Ethel," he drawled.

Well, okay. Lucy and Ethel. The names have stuck. But Lucy and Ethel have an additional piece of system-sense to share with you:

When the home health aides come, hide the silver!

INVESTING IN THE FUTURE

Life with HIV involves surprises and unexpected changes. You can't predict or manage everything. Just when you have your little pie chart all figured out, something unexpected happens. It's like the weather in New England. The bottom line is: Watch out for signs of change. And maintain your flexibility.

You have to put the *living* back into "living with HIV." Being flexible is the first step. Reclaiming your sense of the future is the second. When I asked Rachel how she thinks about the future, here's what she said:

Two things became clear once I got this disease: who I care about, and what I care about. In a nutshell, I care about my daughter and me and creating a life that works for both of us.

That means, first of all, taking care of business so that it won't get in the way. I made up a living will and a real will. I got life insurance and health insurance. And I'm still looking for an individual disability policy, although I have group disability through my job. I still have marriage problems, which I'm working on.

If there is a cure tomorrow, AIDS Action will go away. And I will go to work in the pro-choice movement. I am determined to be around people with whom I feel political affinity.

Right now, I do AIDS work. I like the work environment. There are many reasons for me to be at AIDS Action, not the least of which is that I can be myself. I like that and I'm not giving it up. I couldn't go back to the computer company I worked for before. They don't know the real me — and if they found out they wouldn't like it. At AIDS Action, I can tell the agency director that Earth Shoes are a conspiracy of the Radical Right to make leftists look like assholes and she laughs. I couldn't say that to the vice president of a normal company.

In the meantime, I've started my own business, selling antique costume jewelry. Something new and quite unexpected.

You know how kids ask each other questions like, "If you were going to die soon and you could do anything you wanted, what would you do?" Well, in the spring of 1991, shortly before my thirty-fourth birthday, I was having lunch with an acquaintance. I'd known I was positive for a year. As we chatted, I said, "If I were free to do anything, I would do something with antiques. I've always liked antiques. I'm a collector; I go to shows on weekends. I think I'm going to buy and sell costume jewelry."

This spontaneous remark surprised us both. Later, as I thought it over, I said, "Why not? This is what I do for fun. Why shouldn't I do this for a living? *I want to shop for a living!*"

Now I do. Buying costume jewelry is my second job. So, when I think years into the future, I see myself working in some other progressive cause and selling costume jewelry. And feeling like my life is my own.

■

Rachel and I have dealt with many of the same issues as we reorganized our priorities on account of HIV. Her summary of this process is the best I've ever heard:

I once heard a PWA tell a group, "I've known I had AIDS for eight months and these have been the happiest months of my life." I would not say these have been the happiest two years of my life. They haven't been. I'd give up a lot to get HIV out of my life. But I will say that HIV has forced me to look at my life and get into a better position.

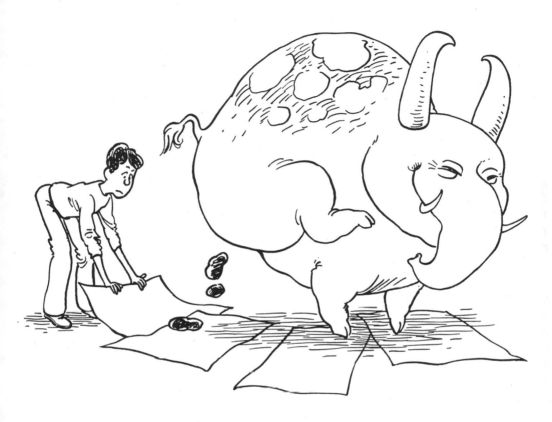

MORAL: **Make room in your life for HIV Business...**
Managing HIV is your number-one priority.

8

Life
Goes On

In July 1991, as Rachel was telling her husband she was HIV-positive and was setting up an HIV conference, I had an unusual visit with my doctor, Millie. It illustrated how much my life had changed since HIV.

It was my monthly appointment. I was relatively healthy. I'd been on ddI almost two years and my lesions had continued to shrink and fade. As ddI was still experimental, we were required to draw blood monthly and send the results to Bristol-Myers.

I was seated in an exam room, waiting for Millie. She walked in and asked, "How are you doing?"

"Great! Nothing wrong."

"Would you mind if one of the new residents examined you today?"

I told her that would be fine.

A few minutes later, the resident, a young woman about twenty-four years old, entered and greeted me.

"I understand you have a KS problem."

"Yes I do, but it's under control now."

She looked at my arm and pointed. "Is that a new lesion?"

"No," I chuckled, "that's a bruise. I've taken up roller-blading recently and had a spill the other day. I'm very careful," I added. "I wear pads and gloves, but I haven't learned how to stop yet. I was zooming down a hill and fell."

"Rollerblading!" she echoed softly as she leafed through my medical history. I knew it showed that I was forty-one and that in 1986 I had been considered disabled and walked with a cane. It also contained numerous accounts of radiation and chemotherapy.

Pad of paper in hand, she made a note to herself.

"By the way," I added, "I need to keep this appointment brief. Just fifteen minutes."

"What's up?"

"Channel 5 is doing a story on how long it takes the FDA to approve new drugs. They're going to interview me! The crew will be back at my house in an hour, so I want to put on something pretty and fluff up my hair."

"Uh-huh." She scribbled. "What else is going on? You look a little tired."

"I'm fine today, but yesterday was exhausting. There was a party for the staff of AIDS Action, hosted by the board of directors, and, as a board member, I volunteered to be the organizer! You won't believe what happened. Do you want to hear the story?"

She nodded.

I continued, breathlessly. "I rented a booze cruise boat with a canopied dance floor and a DJ and food for 120 people. It was marvelous. There was almost a tornado and it was quite exciting."

"Really? Tell me more."

"We were all dancing madly on the top deck, heading towards the outer harbor, when I noticed the wind picking up and a nasty black cloud on the horizon. When the whole sky got ugly, I climbed to the steering cabin and asked the captain, 'At what point do you turn back?'

"'They've issued a gale *watch*,' he told me. 'When they issue a gale *warning*, we head in.' At that very moment, his radio squawked an announcement of a gale warning!

"'Are we heading in?' I asked.

"The captain was frowning as he watched the storm move our way, flashing thunderbolts."

At this point, I saw the student had stopped taking notes altogether and was listening intently. I continued.

"The captain told me, 'This boat doesn't move that fast. At the rate this squall is coming in, we don't have time.'

"I was alarmed. 'What do we do?'

"'I'll head for those islands. They'll provide some shelter.'

"I headed back upstairs as the squall hit. Thunder and lightning! The crowd kept dancing. Sheets of warm rain blew sideways, right across the dance floor. And here's the best part: The DJ put on the theme song to 'Gilligan's Island.' You know, 'Sit right back while I tell you a tale, a tale of a three-hour cruise.' The crowd screamed and danced all the harder.

"The storm lasted half an hour, I had another cocktail, and we got in safely. I had a lot of details to coordinate and we didn't get home until very late. That's why I look a little tired today."

The student seemed lost in thought. I wondered what was going on. I glanced at her notepad and saw that she had written, *Dementia?*

I chuckled to myself and thought, *Let's see what happens next.*

"Would you excuse me for a minute?" she said and stepped out.

A moment later, Millie came in and clucked. "You're torturing her, aren't you?"

"I am not. She asked me questions and I gave her answers!"

Millie rolled her eyes and retreated, shaking her head. The student returned a few moments later and sat down. She looked me in the eye and said evenly, "I've learned a lot today."

That line stuck with me, because I've learned a lot, too. July 1991, was the month I started rollerblading and met this student doctor. At the same time, Michael and I began planning this book. In the back of my mind, I was not sure I'd be healthy enough to finish such a long project. It's been a busy year since then.

THINKING ABOUT WHAT'S NEXT

In April 1992, Michael Connolly and I sat on a porch in Provincetown, looking at the ocean and preparing to edit this text. My health was good — better, in fact, than when we had started.

At the outset I was cautious, even ambivalent. It's difficult for me to make long-term plans and commitments. I can go six months out, maybe a year. I knew the book would be an eighteen-month project, from planning through marketing. A project that long was daunting. I hesitated. I'm glad I chose to go ahead. I would have been angry with myself if I'd let this much time go by without doing something constructive.

My career as a PWA has been a series of projects, each

one a little newer and larger than the last. My first volunteer assignments at AIDS Action used my systems analysis skills. I was the volunteer information systems manager, in 1988. Then I was the agency's unpaid operational director for nine months, in 1989. (It felt more like nine years.) In 1990, I became a board member, focusing on quality of service issues and strategic planning. I was becoming a professional PWA. I spoke with the media about experimental drugs and I sat on many panels about managing your doctor.

"Where do I want to be in five years?" I ask myself that question and I hope you do the same. As I finish this book, I'm wondering about my next project. Will I continue writing? I do have a concept for another book. Perhaps this book has been the seed of a new career.

I know I don't want to spend my time following other people's rules and priorities. I do want to have a life, as my friend Kathy advised in 1986. I want to keep learning, making new friends, and working on projects that stimulate me without stressing my immune system. I also might like to travel, which I haven't done since I was younger. In short, I want to invest in myself.

What can I do to start moving in that direction? That's the second question I'll need to address. In the meantime, Mario and I have taken steps to ensure our financial security. We bought a condo for a price at which he could afford to pay the mortgage, if he had to. That was the essential first step. I don't want to spend my life hemmed in by avoidable crises.

What about you?

What would you like to be doing with your life in five years? Take a few moments to imagine a future that is worth planning for. You can always change your mind.

Let's assume there will be an HIV treatment that will keep you healthy for the next five to ten years. And let's assume that a better treatment will be developed after that — sort of a cure.

- What would you love to be doing?
- Do you already have some of the necessary skills and resources?
- What can you do to begin realizing some of your dreams?
- How will you feel in five years if you're healthy — but have done nothing to develop your life?

There are a lot of stupid systems out there, ready to tell you how to live your life. You can take control. I sincerely hope you do.

MEANWHILE, BACK AT THE RANCH

Last Christmas, I had dinner at Stevie and Jean's. While Stevie puttered in the kitchen, Kelly showed me her karate trophy and demonstrated a few kicks and jabs. While Manny sat on the living room couch, Tommy and I walked into the kitchen, just as Stevie opened the oven, where a ham had been roasting for two hours.

"Jean!" called Stevie. "You forgot to take the plastic off the ham!"

I looked at the pan, dumbfounded. Jean wandered into the kitchen.

"Jean," I asked, "how ever did you glaze the ham — pineapples and all — without taking off the plastic?"

"It was a *very* hectic morning," she sighed. Behind her stood Tommy in the doorway, observing the fuss. He looked at me and raised his eyebrows. I smirked and raised *my* eyebrows, thinking, *At least* his *mother remembers to cook dinner!*

He grinned back.

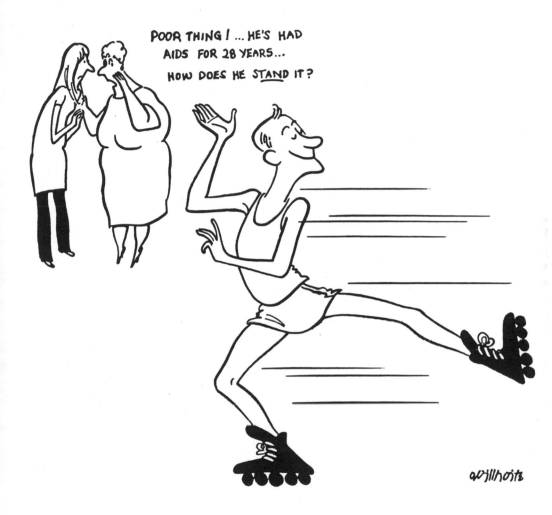

MORAL: **Plan on living, just in case you do!**

Epilogue:
Where Are They Now?

Kathy, who told me to keep living in 1986, is waiting tables in New York to finance her voice lessons. She's launching an opera career — and just invited me to a recital nine months away.

Doc Clean is long gone — wherabouts unknown. I imagine he's putting on a rubber glove somewhere right now.

Julio, the phlebotomist who mislabeled my blood, is notorious among Boston PWAs. A manager at the hospital told me the Lab is being reorganized and Julio has been shunted off to someplace less conspicuous.

Bubbles is still head of Oncology. I haven't had to see him in almost three years.

Clark Kent was the only doctor who supported my attempt to get ddI in 1990. He left the hospital and works with an AIDS research group. He was too good for the system.

Millie is well established at BI. She has twenty-five HIV-infected patients, is a whiz on the computer, and knows how to work the system. After reviewing a draft of this book, she said my memory is quite good. She also said her job requires more analytical skill than I have acknowledged. "If you get sick, you'll see!" she assured me earnestly. After a pause, she added, "That's not a threat! Really!"

Doc Rayon, the Infectious Disease specialist who told me ddI was too risky, is still at Beth Israel. Now a nationally recognized infectious disease specialist, she gets on TV every now and then.

Remember the hospital billing department? My June 1992, hospital bill was a new blue color and a lovely new format — and nine pages long. Someone had carefully used white-out to eliminate over two dozen erroneous charges. The final bill was also whited out and then corrected, in handwritten ink. (It should, you remember, be zero.) It was $298.26. I wonder how long it took to come up with that number? *What a system!*

Larry Killian died in July 1990. We think of him often and know that he is grinning.

Michael Connolly left AIDS Action a few months after Larry died and now consults to non-profit organizations. When not working on this book, he tends the garden begun by his lover, Michael. It has spawned baby gardens up and down his street.

David Aronstein is now the director of education at AIDS Action. He introduced his lover to France on their vacation this year. David and I continue to dine out regularly. He wishes we all lived in Paris.

Rachel is still fundraising and says she is becoming the queen of antique jewelry. Her royal behavior causes comment at work and at home.

Taffy, the advocate who had no idea how to get ddI, left AIDS Action and went to the AIDS Office in the Massachusetts Department of Public Health, where he is director of client services. Taffy visits AIDS organizations and recommends how much they will get funded. There are several contracts out on his head.

Taffy's former boss, Daddy Earl, is now in charge of an adult mental health day care center at a state hospital. *He has the keys.*

My nephew Tommy is eight and his sister Kelly is seven. When I was diagnosed, they were two and one, respectively, and I didn't think I would live long enough for them to remember me. Kelly is becoming a karate master — she's ranked first in her class, nationally. The boys at school give her wide berth. Tommy is quieter than his sister and an excellent student. Tommy and Kelly have an 18-month-old brother, Matthew, who has the best temperament of them all.

My mother died in September 1991. She had many ailments over the years — breast cancer, emphysema, diabetes, glaucoma, and Thorazine-induced Parkinson's disease. Nonetheless, she smoked two packs a day, right to the end. When I received my AIDS diagnosis in 1986, I never thought I would outlive one of my parents.

My father, Manny, has sold the house in which I grew up. My brother Stevie and his wife are selling their house. Together, they have all bought a big house on Cape Cod, where they plan to live happily ever after. Tommy asked if Mario and I would move in. I explained that they don't make houses big enough for all of us!

Afterword

For those of you who particularly enjoyed our systems approach to managing your health care, we have a few final words about managing the bureaucracy as a whole.

Up till now, we have focused on the individual with HIV. Our prescription for living longer by taking control of your life and your treatment is: Know the HIV bureaucracy; get up-to-date treatment information; question authority; and act.

Our advice is based on the assumption that *knowledge is power.* This is true not only at the level of the individual, but also for larger systems. The HIV epidemic is a case in point. Rarely has so much knowledge been available to and used by so many. This constitutes a major difference between HIV and other diseases.

Why is this?

Not because the hospitals, insurance companies, drug companies, or federal government have taken initiative to make information available. Far from it. They have resisted public access and even disregarded the information they have themselves. Neither scientific progress nor government action is responsible for the current availability of HIV information.

Where do people with HIV get their information? From community-based organizations like GMHC, ACT-UP, and Project Inform. Who advocates for the prompt distribution of both information and treatment alternatives? The same groups. These groups have *changed* the health system. A moment's reflection will reveal the reason for their success: *political power.*

HIV differs from other diseases not only in the rapid generation and dissemination of knowledge, but also in the way people with HIV and their supporters have used knowledge to change the system itself.

The HIV community organizations were founded in the early 1980s — years before the federal government first funded HIV research or treatment (1984) and before HIV appeared on the front page of the *New York Times* (1985). These organizations were founded by gay people who recognized the start of a major epidemic — and saw authorities look the other way. The pattern is familiar to every oppressed community in the United States.

The founders of community organizations recognized that HIV was a health crisis with a profoundly political dimension. They got organized, educated people at risk, cared for the sick, and slowly forced the system to change. Today, anyone who wants up-to-date HIV treatment information, including experimental drug treatment data, can get it — *even your doctor.*

Does this mean the institutional battles have been won and individuals need only take advantage of the resources the system offers? Hardly.

Being gay and HIV-positive and living in Boston at the time of the Disabilities Act of 1992 can be compared to being black and living in Mississippi at the time of the Civil Rights Act of 1964. Important legal measures have been taken — but there is a long way to go. Knowing that your landlord may not legally lock you out if you have HIV is not the same as enjoying the free exercise of your rights. *The system is still dysfunctional and needs to be changed.*

As you know, we encourage people to take control of their lives by being active, particularly by volunteering at whatever level is personally rewarding. Volunteer to help sick people. Organize fundraisers for service organizations. Teach safer sex. Write a check. If you are interested in broader system change, join a group to work on one of the goals we've outlined below. Write to your political representatives, or contact the local organization of a political party.

You can make a difference. Please do.

Ten Suggestions for Fixing the HIV System

1. Reform the health insurance system by changing state regulations to:
   - Eliminate pre-existing condition clauses or require insurance companies to cover former policyholders for pre-existing conditions which began while they were still insured;
   - Give gay and unmarried partners access to health insurance via domestic-partners bills;
   - Require insurance companies to pay for experimental drugs;
   - Simplify and standardize billing forms and procedures for all insurance companies and medical facilities.

2. Eliminate the Medicaid spend-down provision, which requires that recipients be destitute.

3. Create anonymous T4 testing programs.

4. Regulate the Medical Information Bureau and enforce existing regulations of insurance companies.

5. Institute a program of universal health insurance. ***This will make suggestions one through four unnecessary.***

6. Change disability insurance procedures to make it easier for people with HIV on disability to work when they want to and feel able to do so, without jeopardizing their disability status.

7. Institute municipal and statewide needle exchange programs and decriminalize needle possession.

8. Give safer-sex education to people as they become sexually active, i.e., in junior high school and high school.

9. Legislate equal rights for lesbian and gay people.

10. Build a better condom.

Appendix:
Getting More Information

These are some leading newsletters of interest to people with HIV:

AIDS Treatment News: Published twice monthly. The cost of a subscription ranges from $45 for those with low incomes to $230 for businesses and professionals. People with AIDS who cannot afford a subscription are encouraged to call. ATN, PO Box 411256, San Francisco, CA 94141. (800) TREAT-1-2 or (415) 255-0588.

BETA: Bulletin of Experimental Treatments for AIDS. Published quarterly by the San Francisco AIDS Foundation. For subscription information call (800) 327-9893.

Project Inform. Serves as a clearinghouse for information about treatments for AIDS. The newsletter, *PI Perspective*, is published quarterly. A $25 tax-deductible donation, which covers future issues, is requested upon receipt of the first newsletter. 347 Dolores Street, Suite 301, San Francisco, CA 94110. (800) 822-7422; in California: (800) 334-7422; in San Francisco: (800) 558-9051.

Treatment Issues. Published ten times a year. Suggested tax-deductible donation ranges from $30 (individuals) to $60 (corporations). GMHC, 129 West 20th St., New York, NY 10011. (212) 337-1950.

Positively Aware. Published monthly. Subscriptions are $25. TPA Network, 1340 West Irving Park, Box 259, Chicago, IL 60613. (312) 404-8726.

Positive Directions News. Published quarterly. Subscriptions $25, or sliding scale for low-income people. Positive Directions, 140 Clarendon Street, Suite 805, Boston, MA 02116. (617) 262-3456.

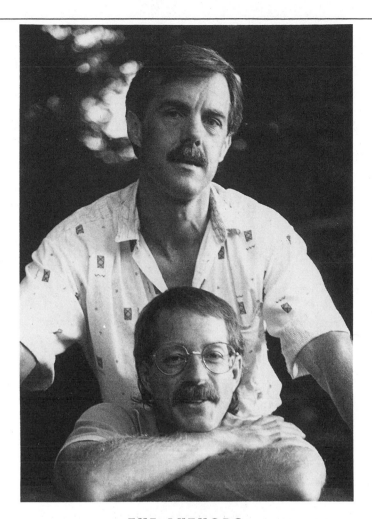

THE AUTHORS:

Michael A. Connolly (standing) has worked with most New England AIDS service organizations as a management consultant. He previously worked with the AIDS Action Committee of Massachusetts. **Robert A. Rimer** (seated; also on the book cover) is a computer analyst and the former deputy executive director of the AIDS Action Committee. As a seven-year AIDS survivor, he is frequently interviewed by the Boston media for HIV-related stories. They both live in the greater Boston area.

How many people do you know who should read

HIV-Positive: Working the System?

The advice in this book can save lives. We encourage you to pass a copy along to a friend when you're done it with, or to get them their own copy. You can purchase copies at bookstores, or by mail, using the order form on the last page.

Special quantity rates
To help disseminate this information more widely, we offer the following bulk discounts for both organizations and individuals:

1–3 copies: $13.00 each
4–9 copies: $12.00 each
10–29 copies: $10.00 each
30–100 copies: $9.00 each

See last page for order form and full instructions.

OTHER ALYSON TITLES
OF INTEREST

THE ALYSON ALMANAC, by Alyson Publications, $9.00. History, biographies, a congressional report card, and scores of useful addresses are collected here.

BI ANY OTHER NAME, edited by Loraine Hutchins and Lani Kaahumanu, $12.00. Over seventy women and men from all walks of life describe their lives as bisexuals.

BROTHER TO BROTHER, edited by Essex Hemphill, $9.00. Fiction, essays, and poetry by black gay men.

COMING OUT RIGHT, by Wes Muchmore and William Hanson, $8.00. A practical guide for the newly out gay man revised for the realities of the 1990s.

THE FIRST GAY POPE, by Lynne Yamaguchi Fletcher, $8.00. Hundreds of achievements, records, and firsts are recorded in this entertaining new reference.

THE GAY BOOK OF LISTS, by Leigh Rutledge, $9.00. A fascinating compilation of gay history, personalities, and trivia.

GOLDENBOY, by Michael Nava, $9.00. Henry Rios thought his client was guilty. He took the case anyway. Those were merely his first two mistakes.

A LOTUS OF ANOTHER COLOR, edited by Rakesh Ratti, $10.00. Gay men and lesbians from India, Pakistan, and other South Asian countries tell their stories.

SOCIETY AND THE HEALTHY HOMOSEXUAL, by George Weinberg, $8.00. The man who coined the term *homophobia* tells gay people how to guard against its subtle influence.

THE TROUBLE WITH HARRY HAY, by Stuart Timmons, $13.00. A colorful and original American life reflects the growth of the gay liberation movement.

UNNATURAL QUOTATIONS, by Leigh W. Rutledge, $9.00. Quotations by, for, or about gay men and lesbians.

SUPPORT YOUR LOCAL BOOKSTORE

Most of the books described above are available at your
nearest gay or feminist bookstore, and many of them will be
available at other bookstores. If you can't get these books
locally, order by mail using this form.

Enclosed is $_____ for the following books. (Add $1.00
postage when ordering just one book. If you order two or
more, we'll pay the postage.)

Qty.   **Title**   **Total Price**

_____   _____   _____

_____   _____   _____

_____   _____   _____

_____   _____   _____

_____   _____   _____

_____   _____   _____

                                            Order Total _____

name: _____

address: _____

city: _____ state: _____ zip: _____

ALYSON PUBLICATIONS
Dept. I-8, 40 Plympton St., Boston, MA 02118

After June 30, 1994, please write for current catalog.